Pharmaceutics II
Including Practicals

for Second Year Diploma in Pharmacy

Based on Syallabus Prescribed by PCI
Course Regulations, 1991

Pharmaceutics II

Including Practicals

for Second Year Diploma in Pharmacy

Based on Syallabus Prescribed by PCI
Course Regulations, 1991

Gaurav Agarwal

MPharm (BITS-Pilani) PhD

Dean, Faculty of Pharmacy
RP Indraprastha Institute of Technology
Karnal, Haryana

CBS

CBS Publishers & Distributors Pvt Ltd

New Delhi • Bengaluru • Chennai • Kochi • Kolkata • Mumbai
Hyderabad • Jharkhand • Nagpur • Patna • Pune • Uttarakhand

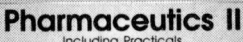

Pharmaceutics II
Including Practicals

for Second Year Diploma in Pharmacy

ISBN: 978-93-88178-90-7

Copyright © Author and Publisher

First Edition: 2019

Reprint: 2019, 2021 **2024**

Published by Satish Kumar Jain and Produced by Varun Jain for

CBS Publishers & Distributors Pvt Ltd

4819/XI Prahlad Street, 24 Ansari Road, Daryaganj, New Delhi 110 002, India
Ph: 011-23289259, 23266861, 23266867   Website: www.cbspd.com
Fax: 011-23243014   e-mail: delhi@cbspd.com; cbspubs@airtelmail.in
Corporate Office: 204 FIE, Industrial Area, Patparganj, Delhi 110 092
Ph: 011-4934 4934   Fax: 011-4934 4935   e-mail: publishing@cbspd.com;
                                              publicity@cbspd.com

Branches

- **Bengaluru:** Seema House 2975, 17th Cross, K.R. Road, Banasankari 2nd Stage, Bengaluru 560 070, Karnataka
  Ph: +91-80-26771678/79   Fax: +91-80-26771680   e-mail: bangalore@cbspd.com
- **Chennai:** 7, Subbaraya Street, Shenoy Nagar, Chennai 600 030, Tamil Nadu
  Ph: +91-44-26680620, 26681266   Fax: +91-44-42032115   e-mail: chennai@cbspd.com
- **Kochi:** 42/1325, 1326, Power House Road, Opp. KSEB, Power House, Ernakulam 682018, Kochi, Kerala
  Ph: +91-484-4059061-65   Fax: +91-484-4059065   e-mail: kochi@cbspd.com
- **Kolkata:** No. 6/B, Ground Floor, Rameswar Shaw Road, Kolkata 700014 (West Bengal), India
  Ph: +91-33-2289-1126, 2289-1127, 2289-1128   e-mail: kolkata@cbspd.com
- **Mumbai:** PWD Shed, Gala No. 25/26, Ramchandra Bhatt Marg, Next to JJ Hospital, Gate No. 2 Opp. Union Bank of India, Noorbaug, Mumbai 400009, Maharashtra, India
  Ph: +91-22-66661880/89   e-mail: mumbai@cbspd.com

Representatives

- **Hyderabad** 0-9885175004   - **Jharkhand** 0-9811541605   - **Nagpur** 0-9421945513
- **Patna** 0-9334159340   - **Pune** 0-9623451994   - **Uttarakhand** 0-9716462459

Printed at Glorious Printers, Jhilmil Industrial Area, Delhi, India

to
my loving kids
Shreya
and
Vaidish

Preface

This book *Pharmaceutics II* is designed specifically as per PCI (Pharmacy Council of India) for D Pharmacy second year students. It contains a comprehensive description, an overview of existing knowledge of pharmaceutics and making it appropriate for introductory and institutional purposes.

Being an interdisciplinary subject, it is today covering a wide range of interest both among the students and teaching communities. Taking this increasing interest into account, this book gives a comprehensives introduction to the subject. The text not only deals with the basic concepts but also emphasizes technical and practical aspects of the subject. The book is primarily intended as text for students of pharmacy for degree and diploma courses.

The book contains numerous specimens, vivid illustrations, tables, diagrams and flow diagrams to present the ideas. The distinguishing feature is ample question bank at the end of the book. The structure and the content of the book have changed to reflect modern thinking and current university curricula throughout the world. The distinguishing feature is practical related to subject at the end of the book. In spite of great care there might be some mistakes and deficiencies. I will be grateful for giving suggestions to improve upon myself. So go through the content and do mail to me at gbitsian@rediffmail.com.

Gaurav Agarwal

Acknowledgments

It is a moment of great pleasure and immense satisfaction for me to express deep gratitude and gratefulness to Proff. (Dr) Gajendra Singh, Dean, Faculty of Pharmaceutical Sciences, Pt BD Sharma university of health sciences, Rohtak for inspiring me to bring out this book.

I am specially thankful to Shri RP Singal Ji Chairman, RP Educational trust, for his all time support and encouragement.

My special thanks to Er Bharat Singal, Secertary, RP Educational Trust for inspiring us to bring out this book.

I am indebted to Dr Rajiv Singal (Vice Chairman) RP Educational Trust, Dr Saurabh Gupta and Shri DL Mittal, RPIIT Technical and Medical Campus, for their motivation.

Special thanks to my peers Ritesh Srivastav (Training and Placement Head) for his moral support.

I express my gratefulness to Shri YN Arjuna, Senior Vice President-Publishing, CBS Publishers & Distributors and especial thanks to Shri Satish K Jain Proprietor CBS Publishers & Distributors for his sincere efforts.

I express my gratitude to my Father Er VK Agarwal and my mother Asha Agarwal for there all time blessings and moral support.

Last but not least, I express my love to my wife Shilpi for her all of in-spite of to inspiration, and dedication. She is always a constant source to motivation in bring out this achievement!

To our numerous students, whom I cannot possibly name individually, I thanks for their class interactions which have been the guiding spirit in selection of the subject matter and its logical arrangement.

Gaurav Agarwal

Contents

Chapter 1

Prescription

"A medical prescription is an order (often in written form) by a qualified health care professional to a pharmacist or other therapist for a treatment to be provided to their patient".

A prescription is a legal document which not only instructs in the preparation and provision of the medicine or device but indicates the prescriber takes responsibility for the clinical care of the patient and the outcomes that may or may not be achieved.

R$_x$

There are various theories about the origin of this symbol—some note its similarity to the eye of Horus, others to the ancient symbol for Jupiter, both gods whose protection may have been sought in medical contexts. Alternatively, it may be intended as an abbreviation of the Latin "recipe", the imperative form of "recipere", "to take", and it is quite possible that more than one of these factors influenced its form. Literally, "Recipe" means simply "Take...." and when a doctor writes a prescription beginning with "R$_x$", he or she is completing the command. This was probably originally directed at the pharmacist who needed to take a certain amount of each ingredient to compound the medicine, rather than at the patient who must "take" the medicine, in the sense of consuming it. The word "prescription" can be decomposed into "pre" and "script" and literally means, "to write before" a drug.

1

PARTS OF A PRESCRIPTION

Prescriptions are generally written on a typical format which is usually kept as pads. A typical prescription consists of the following parts:

1. **Physician (Prescriber) Information:** It is essential so that the doctor could be contacted in emergency to seek clarification and necessary instruction, missing words, confirmation, etc. Following information is mentioned on the prescription:
   i. Doctor's name, designation and Registration Number
   ii. Address with phone number and e-mail.
   iii. Date of issue of prescription.
   iv. Prescription number, (required when calling the pharmacy for a refill or for medical claim Purposes).

2. **Patient Information:** The name, address, age and sex of the patient help in identifying the prescription. Date of prescribing and date(s) of presentation for filling are necessary for keeping accurate records and ascertaining the needs of the patient. Age and sex of the patient, if mentioned, help the pharmacist to check the prescribed dose(s) of the medication.

3. **Superscription:** The superscription which consists of the heading where the symbol R_x (an abbreviation for recipe, the Latin for 'take thou' or 'you take' is found. R_x symbol comes before the inscription. The sign at the foot of the letter R is believed to represent the sign of Jupiter, the God of Healing. Some historians believe that the symbol R_x originated from the sign of Jupiter.

4. **Inscription:** The inscription (body of prescription) comprises an important part of prescription containing:
   i. Name(s) of drug(s) and their quantities,
   ii. Other chief ingredients of the prescription with quantity,
   iii. Instruction regarding dosage form like tablet, capsule, suspension, mixture, etc. and
   iv. Dose and quantity of prescription

5. **Subscription:** The subscription gives specific directions for the pharmacist on how to compound the medication. Most of direction is usually expressed in contracted Latin or in the form of abbreviation. Instructions for preparation are

also given such as: 'make a mixture', 'mix and make 10 tablets', or 'dispense 10 tablets'.

6. **Signatura:** The signatura which gives instructions to the patient. These instructions are preceded by abbreviation 'Sig.' from the Latin, meaning 'mark.' The signatura should always be written in English; however, physicians continue to insert Latin abbreviations, e.g. '1 cap tid pc' which the pharmacist translates into English as 'take one capsule three times daily after meals'. It may also contain special instructions, warnings, followed by the signature of the prescriber.

7. **Renewal:** The number of times a prescription is to be repeated, is written by the physician under renewal instructions.

8. **Signature:** Finally, the prescription must bear the signature of the prescriber to impart it the legal validity.

9. **Other important instructions:**
   a. Qty: "Quantity" or how much is in the package.
   b. Mfg.: "Manufacturer" or who makes the medication.
   c. Expiry date: When the drug is going to expire.
   d. Take complete/full course: Means that patient should finish taking the entire contents of the prescription even if feeling better especially patient taking antibiotics. This is to avoid recurrence of infection and development of resistance.
   e. Take with/without food: Means whether the medication is to be taken after a meal or empty stomach. Some medications work better when the stomach is full while some medications work better when the stomach is empty.
   f. Take four times a day: Means to take the medication four times in 24 hours with equal spacing of time. It is different than 'Take every four hours'. If any confusion occurs when to give the medications, one should consult doctor or pharmacist. Most medications do not have to be precisely timed to be effective, but some do.
   g. Take as needed as symptoms persist: Means the medication can be taken when symptoms are present, without consulting the prescriber.

h. The package may also have bright colored warning labdls with additional information. The following are examples:
  i. Safe storage instructions, such as 'keep refrigerated'.
  ii. Instructions for use, such as 'shake well before use'.
  iii. Possible side effects, such as 'may cause drowsiness'.

The use of Latin in prescription writing is traditional (Fig. 1.1). Although teaching of Latin has slowly gone out of the curricula of medicine and pharmacy, some of the words and abbreviations have very deep roots and physicians still use them frequently. In earlier days, a prescription was a secret between the physician and the pharmacist and a mystery for the patient. With the increasing awareness about drugs no secrecy is now warranted. As such the patient has a right to know what medication has been prescribed and his interest is protected under the Consumer Protection Act.

Handling of Prescription

The following procedure should be adopted by the pharmacist while handling the prescription for compounding and dispensing (Fig. 1.1):

1. Receiving
2. Reading and checking

AGARWAL NURSING HOME
Khatghar, Quila, Bareilly Ph: 0581-2514560

Date: 28-2-08

Name: Mr. Ashish Agarwal　　Age: 19 Yrs　　Sex: Male
Address: 51, Parvez Coloney, Bareilly.
Rx (Superscription)

(Inscription)	Sodium bicarbonate	3 g
	Compound tincture of cardamon	2 ml
	Simple synup	6 ml
	Water qs	90 ml

Fiat mistura (Subscription)
Sig. Cochleare magnum ter in die post cibos sumenda. (Signatura)

Refill: _____

Sd/-
Dr.S.K.Agarwal
MBBS, MD
Regd. No. 14328

Fig. 1.1: A typical prescription

3. Collecting and weighing the materials
4. Compounding, labeling and packaging.

MODERN METHODS OF PRESCRIBING

Nowadays, the majority of the drugs are available in the market as ready-made formulations manufactured by different pharmaceutical companies. There is no need to dispense the drugs by the pharmacist. In the present days, the role of pharmacist is to hand over the ready-made preparations to the patients and provide advice if demanded regarding its mode of administration, dose schedule, drug interactions and adverse reactions, etc. The practice of writing long, complicated prescriptions containing several ingredients, adjuvants or, vehicles is not required.

In the present day set up, the writing of prescription is more significant. The prescription should be precise, accurate, clear and easily readable. As far as possible, the Latin terms should be avoided. In olden days the Latin language was used to conceal certain facts from the patient. But nowadays, the prescriptions are written in English language and dose is prescribed in metric system for the convenience of the patients.

The drugs should be prescribed by their official (generic) name and not by proprietary or trade name. There are certain advantages and disadvantages of prescribing the drugs by proprietary names, which are as under.

Advantages

i. It is easy to remember proprietary names because they are very catchy, e.g., Librium (chlordiazepoxide), Calmpose (diazepam), and Crocin (paracetamol).
ii. It is easy to communicate with the patient.
iii. The continuity can be maintained by prescribing the same proprietary name every time.
iv. The bioavailability of drugs changed with the change of adjuvants used in drug formulations manufactured by different manufacturers. So, only those proprietary drugs can be prescribed which have a better bioavailability.

Disadvantages

   i. It is cheaper to prescribe the drugs by their official names.

   ii. It becomes difficult for a pharmacist to dispense the substitute of the drug which is available in the stock.

There are four types of prescriptions which are generally received by the retail drug store:

1. Prescription in general practice
2. Private prescriptions
3. Hospital prescriptions meant for 'outpatients'
4. Hospital prescriptions meant for 'inpatients'.

A typical modern prescription is shown below (Fig. 1.2).

LEGALITY OF PRESCRIPTION

Prescriptions, when handwritten, are notorious for being often illegible 5% according to an Irish study. Contrary to popular belief, pharmacists do not have special deciphering skills. When in doubt, they call the doctor. At other times, even though some of the individual letters are illegible, the position of the legible letters and length of the word is sufficient to distinguish the medication based on the knowledge of the pharmacist (Fig. 1.2).

AGARWAL NURSING HOME
Khatghar, Bareilly
Tel.: 0581-2514530 Mob:09259082272

Date: 20-1-08

Name: Mrs. Tanvi Agarwal   Age: 21 Yrs   Sex: Female
Address: 55, Parvez Coloney, Bareilly.
R_X

Cap. Ampicillin   500 mg
Dispense 20 capsules.
One capsule to be taken with water four times a day for five days.

Sd/-
Refill: _____   Dr. Abhinav Agarwal
MBBS, MD
Regd. No. 0122345

Fig. 1.2: Modern form of prescription

Writing Good Prescription

Following are some tips for writing good prescription:
1. Careful use of decimal points to avoid ambiguity.
2. Avoid unnecessary decimal points: 5 ml instead of 5.0 ml to avoid possible misinterpretation of 5.0 = 50
3. Always zero prefix decimals: e.g. 0.5 instead of .5 to avoid misinterpretation with .5 = 5.
4. Avoid decimals altogether by changing the units: 0.5 g = 500 mg.
5. "ml" is used instead of "cc" or "cm³" even though they are technically equivalent.
6. Quantities can be given directly or implied by the frequency and duration of the direction.
7. Where possible, usage directions should specify times (7 am, 3 pm, 11 pm) rather than simply frequency (3 times a day) and especially relationship to meals for orally consumed medication.

PHARMACEUTICAL CALCULATIONS

To have a complete understanding of various types calculations, which are involved in dispensing, it is desirable that the pharmacist should have a thorough knowledge regarding weights and measures which are used in calculations.

There are two systems of weights and measures:
1. The imperial system
2. The metric system

Table 1.1: Partial lists of prescription abbreviations

Abbreviation	Latin	Meaning
aa	ana	of each
ad	Ad	up to
ac	ante cibum	before meals
ad	aurio dextra	right ear
ad lib	Ad libitum	use as much as one desires; freely
admov	admove	apply
agit	agita	stir/shake

(Contd.)

Table 1.1: Partial lists of prescription abbreviations *(Contd.)*

Abbreviation	Latin	Meaning
alt h	alternis horis	every other hour
am	ante meridiem	morning, before noon
amp		ampule
amt		amount
aq	aqua	water
al, as	aurio laeva, aurio sinister	left ear
ATC		around the clock
au	auris utrae	both ears
bis	bis	twice
bid	bis in die	twice daily
BM		bowel movement
bol	bolus	as a large single dose (usually intravenously)
BS		blood sugar
BSA		body surface areas
cap, caps	capsula	capsule
c	cum	with (usually written with a bar on top of the "c")
c	cibos	food
cc	cum cibos	with food, (but also cubic centimetre)
cf		with food
comp		compound
cr, crm		cream
D5W		dextrose 5% solution (sometimes written as D5W)
D5NS		dextrose 5% in normal saline (0.9%)
DAW		dispense as written
dc, D/C, disc		discontinue
dieb alt	diebus alternis	every other day
dil		dilute
disp		dispense
div		divide
dtd	dentur tales doses	give of such doses
DW		distilled water
elix		elixir

(Contd.)

Table 1.1: Partial lists of prescription abbreviations *(Contd.)*

Abbreviation	Latin	Meaning
emp	Ex modo prescripto	as directed
emuls	emulsum	emulsion
et	Et	and
ex aq	Ex aqua	in water
fl, fld		fluid
ft	fiat	make; let it be made
g		gram
gr		grain
gtt(s)	gutta(e)	drop(s)
H		hypodermic
h, hr	hora	hour
hs	hora somni	at bedtime
ID		intradermal
IM		intramuscular (with respect to injections)
inj	injectio	injection
IP		intraperitoneal
IV		intravenous
IVP		intravenous push
IVPB		intravenous piggyback
LAS		label as such
LCD		coal tar solution
lin	linimentum	liniment
liq	liquor	solution
lot		lotion
M	misce	mix
m, min	minimum	a minimum
mcg		microgram
mEq		milliequivalent
mg		milligram
mist	mistura	mix
mitte	mitte	send
ml		millilitre
nebul	nebula	a spray
NMT		not more than
noct	nocte	at night

(Contd.)

Table1.1: Partial lists of prescription abbreviations *(Contd.)*

Abbreviation	Latin	Meaning
non rep	non repetatur	no repeats
NS		normal saline (0.9%)
1/2NS		half normal saline (0.45%)
NTE		not to exceed
o_2		both eyes, sometimes written as o2
od	oculus dexter	right eye
os	oculus sinister	left eye
ou	oculus uterque	both eyes
oz		ounce
per	per	by or through
pc	post cibum	after meals
pm	post meridiem	evening or afternoon
prn	pro re nata	as needed
po	per os	by mouth or orally
pr		by rectum
pulv	pulvis	powder
q	quaque	every
q ad	quoque alternis die	every other day
q am	quaque die ante meridiem	everyday before noon
q h	quaque hora	every hour
q hs	quaque hora somni	every night at bedtime
q 1h	quaque 1 hora	every 1 hour; (can replace "1" with other numbers)
qd	quaque die	every day
qid	quater in die	four times a day
qod		every other day
qqh	quater quaque hora	every four hours
qs	quantum sufficiat	a sufficient quantity
R		rectal
rep, rept.	repetatur	repeats
RL, R/L		Ringer's lactate

(Contd.)

Table 1.1: Partial lists of prescription abbreviations *(Contd.)*

Abbreviation	Latin	Meaning
s	sine	without (usually written with a bar on top of the "s")
sa	secundum artum	use your judgement
SC, subc, subq, subcut		subcutaneous
sig		write on label
SL		sublingually, under the tongue
sol	solutio	solution
sos, si op. sit	si opus sit	if there is a need
ss	semis	one half
stat	statim	immediately
supp	suppositorium	suppository
susp		suspension
syr	syrupus	syrup
tab	tabella	tablet
tal, t	talus	such
tbsp		tablespoon
troche	trochiscus	lozenge
tsp		teaspoon
tid	Ter in die	three times a day
tds	Ter die sumendum	three times a day
tiw		three times a week
top		topical
TPN		total parenteral nutrition
tr, tinc, tinct		tincture
ud, ut dict	ut dictum	as directed
ung	unguentum	ointment
USP		United States Pharmacopoeia
vag		vaginally
w		with
w/o		without
X		Times
YO		Years old

1. The Imperial System

Measurement of weights in imperial system: Weight is a measure of the gravitational force acting on a body and is directly proportional to its mass. The imperial system is divided into two parts for the purpose of measurement of weight. These are:

1. Avoirdupois System
2. Apothecaries System

Avoirdupois System: In this system the pound is the standard unit for weighting and all measures of mass are derived from the Imperial Standard Pound (Lb) (Table 1.2).

Apothecaries System: This system is also known as Troy system. The grain is the standard weight in this system and all other weights are derived from it (Table 1.3).

Measurement of capacity in imperial system: The standard units for capacity is the same in both avoirdupois and apothecaries systems. The 'gallon' is the standard unit and all other measurements of capacity are derived it (Table 1.4).

Table 1.2: Avoirdupois system for measurement		
1Lb	=	16 oz (avoir)
1Lb	=	7000 grains
1oz (avoir)	=	7000/16 grains
	=	437.5 grains

Table 1.3: Apothecaries system for measurement		
20 grains	=	1 scruple (Ꝫ)
60 grains	=	1 drachm (ʒ)
480 grains	=	1 ounces (ʒ) (apothe)
8 drachms	=	1 ounces (apothe)
12 ounces	=	1 pound (Lb)
5760 grains	=	1 pound (apothe)

Table 1.4: Measurement of capacity in imperial system		
1 gallon (c)	=	160 fluid ounces
1/4th of a gallon	=	1 quart
1/8th of a gallon	=	1 pint (o)
1/160 of a gallon	=	1 fl ounce (℥)
1/8th of a fl ounce	=	1 fl drachm (℈)
1/60th of fl drachm	=	1 minim (m)
1quart	=	40 fl ounces
1pint	=	20 fl ounces
1 fl ounces	=	480 minims
1fl drachm	=	60 minims

2. The Metric System

The metric system is used in Indian Pharmacopoeia for the measurement of weight and capacity. The metric system in India was implemented from 1st April, 1964 in pharmacy profession.

Measurement of weights in metric system: A 'kilogram' is the standard unit for measurement of weight and all other units are derived from it (Table 1.5) .

Measurement of capacity: A 'liter' is the standard unit for measurement of capacity and all measurements of capacity are derived from it.

1 liter (lt) = 1000 milliliters (ml)

Conversion Tables

The Pharmacopoeia of India (IP) uses only metric system in formulae, but the prescriptions are still written in the Imperial system by many an old time physician's. So a conversion table (given below) is used by pharmacists (Tables 1.6 and 1.7).

PERCENTAGE PREPARATIONS

Many of the prescriptions received in the pharmacy have the amounts of active ingredients expressed as percentage strengths. The physician knows that each active ingredient,

Table 1.5: Measurement as per metric system

1 kilogram (kg)	= 1000 grams
1 hectogarm (hg)	= 100 grams
1 decagram (dag)	= 10 grams
1 decigram (dg)	= 10^{-1} gram
1 centigram (cg)	= 10^{-2} gram
1 miligram (mg)	= 10^{-3} gram
1 microgram (μg or mcg)	= 10^{-6} gram
1 gram (g)	= 1000 mg

when given in certain percentage strength, gives the desired therapeutic effect. Instead of the physician calculating the amount of each ingredient needed for the prescription, he will simply indicate the percentage strength desired for each ingredient and expect the pharmacy to calculate the amount of each ingredient based on its percentage strength.

There are no percentage weights for a torsion balance or percentage graduations on a graduate. The percentage values on a prescription must be changed to amounts which can be weighed (grams) or to amounts, which can be measured (milliliters).

Table 1.6: Conversion tables

i. Weight measures

1kilogram (kg)	=	2.2 lb (pound)
30 g	=	1 ounces (ℨ)
450 g (avoir)	=	1 pound
1 g	=	15 grains
60 mg	=	1 grain

ii. Capacity measures

1000 ml	=	1quart
500 ml	=	1 pint
30 ml	=	1 fluid ounces
4 ml	=	1 fluid drachm
1 ml	=	15 minims
0.06 ml	=	1 minims

Table 1.7: Conversion table for domestic measures

Domestic measure	Metric system	Imperial system
1 drop	0.06 ml	1 minim
1 teaspoonful	4.00 ml	1 fluid drachm
1 dersert spoonful	8.00 ml	2 fluid drachm
1 tablespoonful	15.00 ml	4 fluid drachm
2 tablespoonful	30.00 ml	1 fluid ounce
1 wine glassful	60.00 ml	2 fluid ounce
1 teacupful	120.00 ml	4 fluid ounce
1 tumbler full	240.00 ml	8 fluid ounce

Types of Percent

The term percent means "parts per hundred" and is expressed in the following manner:

1. **w/w Percent:** Weight/Weight percent is defined as the number of grams in 100 g (q.s) of a solid preparation.

   Example: A 5% (w/w) boric acid ointment would contain 5 g of boric acid in each 100 g (q.s) of boric acid ointment.

   Example: A 3% (w/w) vioform powder would contain 3 g of vioform in every 100 g (q.s) of the vioform powder.

2. **w/v percent:** It is defined as the number of grams in 100 milliliters (q.s) of solution.

   Example: A 10% (w/v) potassium chloride (KCL) elixir would contain 10 g of potassium chloride in every 100 milliliters (q.s) of KC1 elixir.

   Example: A 5% (w/v) phenobarbital elixir would contain 5 g of phenobarbital in every 100 milliliters (q.s) of phenobarbital elixir.

3. **v/v percent:** It is defined as the number of milliliters in every 100 ml (q.s) of solution.

   Example: A 70% (v/v) alcoholic solution would contain 70 milliliters of alcohol in every 100 ml (q.s) of solution.

   Example: A 0.5% (v/v) glacial acetic acid solution would contain 0.5 milliliters of glacial acetic acid in each 100 milliliters (q.s) of solution.

4. v/w percent: It is defined as the volume in milliliters of a substance in 100 g (q.s) of solution.

For example, a 10% (v/w) alcoholic solution would contain 10 milliliters of alcohol in every 100 g (q.s) of quantity sufficient solution.

When the type of percent is not stated, it is understood that dilutions are:

1. For dry ingredient in a dry preparation is percent w/w

2. For dry ingredients in a liquid are percent w/v

3. For a liquid in a liquid is percent v/v.

ALCOHOL DILUTION

Dilute alcohols are prepared from 95% alcohol which contains 95 ml of ethyl alcohol and 5 ml of purified water quantity sufficient. When alcohol is mixed with water, the following changes take place:

1. Rise in temperature.

2. Contraction in volume.

3. There is turbid appearance in the solution, because solubility of air is more in alcohol than in water. When alcohol is diluted with water, minute bubbles of air get evolved and make turbid appearance. When alcohol is diluted with water, it is necessary to cool the mixture to about 20°C and then final volume is made up. The formula used is:

Volume of stronger alcohol to be used

$$= \frac{\text{Volume required} \times \text{percentage required}}{\text{Percentage used}}$$

Example: Calculate the amount of 95% alcohol required to prepare 200 ml of 45% alcohol.

Calculation:

Volume required = 200 ml

Percentage of alcohol required = 45

Percentage of alcohol used = 95

By applying the formula:

Volume of stronger alcohol to be used

$$= \frac{\text{Volume required} \times \text{percentage required}}{\text{Percentage used}}$$

$$= \frac{200 \times 45}{95}$$

$$= 1800/19$$

$$= 94.7 \text{ ml}$$

$$\approx 95 \text{ ml (approx.)}$$

95 ml of 95% alcohol is diluted with water to produce 200 ml of 45% dilute alcohol.

Example: Calculate the volume of 95% alcohol required to produce 300 ml of 60% alcohol.

Calculation:

Volume required = 300 ml
Percentage of alcohol required = 60
Percentage of alcohol used = 95

By applying formula:

Volume of stronger alcohol to be used

$$= \frac{\text{Volume required} \times \text{percentage required}}{\text{Percentage used}}$$

$$= \frac{200 \times 45}{95}$$

$$= 18000/95$$

$$= 189.47 \text{ ml}$$

$$\approx 190 \text{ ml (approx.)}$$

190 ml 95% alcohol is diluted with water to produce 300 ml 60% dilute alcohol.

Example: Calculate the quantity of sodium chloride required to prepare 400 ml of a 0.9% solution.

Calculation:

1% w/v solution means 1 g in 100 ml

Hence to prepare 400 ml (0.9%), sodium chloride required is

$$= \frac{0.9 \times 400}{100}$$

with solvent to produce 400 ml makes 0.9% w/v = 3.6 g

Hence 3.6 g of sodium chloride is dissolved in water to produce 400 ml makes 0.9% w/v solution.

Example: Prepare 400 ml of a 5% solution and from 2 L of solution having concentration 1 in 2,000?

Calculation:

Strength of concentrate solution = 5%

Strength of dilute solution = 1 in 2000

$$= 1/2000$$
$$= 0.05\%$$

By applying formula

Degree of dilution = Strength of concentrate/Strength of dilute solution

$$= 5/0.05$$
$$= 100 \text{ times}$$

Volume of the solution to be prepared = 2 L = 2,000 ml

Hence dilute solution is obtained by diluting 2,000/100 = 20 ml of concentrate solution to 2 litre.

Example: Prepare 500 ml of a 1 in 400 solution from the 1 in 800 solution.

Calculation:

Strength of concentrate 1 in 800 = 100/800 = 0.125%

Strength of dilute solution 1 in 4000 = 100/400 = 0.0025%

By applying formula:

Degree of dilution = Strength of concentrate/Strength of dilute solution

$$= 0.125/0.0025$$
$$= 50 \text{ times}$$

Volume of solution to be prepared = 500 ml

Hence dilute solution is obtained by diluting 500/50 = 10 ml of 1 in 800 solution to 500 ml.

Dilution Method for Stock Preparations

In order to make formulation and preparation, the stock solution is diluted especially when the amount required is so small that it cannot be accurately weighed on a torsion balance. Since, it is easier to measure an amount of stock solution than to weigh the ingredients.

Formulas Used

a. Volumes and weights must be expressed in the same units.

b. Concentrations must be expressed in the same units.

c. Formula: V1 C1 = V2 C2

V1 = Volume of stock preparation	C1 = Concentration of stock preparation
V2 = Volume of desired preparation	C2 = Concentration of desired preparation

d. Formula: W1 C1 = W2 C2

W1 = Weight of stock preparation	C1 = Concentration of stock preparation
W2 = Weight of desired preparation	C2 = Concentration of desired preparation

Example: How many milliliters of a 4% stock solution of potassium permanganate (KMnO₄) would be needed to compound 120 ml of 0.02% solution of KMnO₄?

Calculation:

Using the formula.

$$V1\ C1 = V2\ C2$$

Substituting the values

(X) (4%) = (120 ml) (0.02%)

Checking the units and solving

a. Units of concentration are both%.

b. X will have the same units as the volume (i.e. ml)

$$4\ X = 2.4$$

$$X = 0.6\ ml$$

Example: How many grams of 15% zinc oxide ointment can be made from one pound of 20% zinc oxide ointment?

Calculation:

Using the formula

$$W1\ C1 = W2\ C2$$

Substituting the values and solving

$$(X)\ (15\%) = (454\ g)\ (20\%)$$

Note: 1 lb = 454 g

$$15\ X = 9080\ X$$

$$= 605\ g\ or\ 1.33\ lb$$

Example: How many milliliters of 10% povidone iodine (Betadine) solutio0n would be needed to make 2 liters of a 1:2000 Betadine solution?

Calculation:

Using the formula

$$V_1 C_1 = V_2 C_2$$

Substituting the values

$$(X) (10\%) = (2L) (1/2000)$$

Checking the units and solving

  a. Units of concentration of both are not in%.

  b. X will have the same units as the volume (i.e. L)

Converting 10%, it will be 10/100

Now substituting and solving

$$(X).10/100 = (2).(1/2000)$$

$$X = 0.01L \text{ or } 10 \text{ ml}$$

Example: How many milliliters of a 1:200 copper sulphate solution would be needed to make 2000 ml of a 1:4000 solution?

Calculation:

$$V_1 C_1 = V_2 C_2$$

$$(X) (1/200) = (2000 \text{ ml}) (1/4000)$$

$$20 X = 2000 \text{ ml}$$

$$X = 100 \text{ ml}$$

PRACTICE QUESTIONS

1. How many milliliters of a 6% hydrogen peroxide solution would be needed to make 120 ml of 1% hydrogen peroxide solution?

2. How many milliliters of a 10% copper sulphate solution would be needed to make 60 ml of a 2% potassium copper sulphate solution?

3. How many milliliters of a 1:1000 cetrizine HCl solution are needed to make 90 ml of 1:5000 solution?

4. How many milliliters of a 1:50 stock solution should be used to prepare one liter of a 1:4000 solution?

5. How many milliliters of a 2.5% stock solution of a chemical should be used to make 5 liters of a 1:1500 solution?

6. How many milliliters of a 1:200 stock solution should be used to make 120 ml of a 0.025% solution?

7. How many milliliters of a 1:50 stock solution should be used to make 1L of a 0.02% solution?

8. How many milliliters of 10% (W/W) rose water can be made from 450 milliliters of 28% rose water?

9. How many gallons of 60% (V/V) alcohol can be made from 10 gallons of 95% (V/V) alcohol?

10. How many grams of 2% ammoniated mercury ointment can be made from 12.5 grams of 5% ammoniated mercury ointment?

11. How many grams of 10% Betadine ointment can be made from 5 lbs. Of 15% Betadine ointment?

12. How many grams of zinc oxide are needed to make 24 grams of a 4% (w/w) zinc oxide ointment?

13. How many milliliters of a 5% (w/v) boric acid solution can be made from 10 grams of boric acid?

14. How many milliliters of paraldehyde are needed to make 120 ml of a 20% (v/v) paraldehyde solution?

15. How many grams of ephedrine sulfate are needed to make 120 ml of a 2% (w/v) ephedrine sulfate solution?

16. How many grams of boric acid are needed to make 200 ml of a 5% (w/v) boric acid solution?

17. How many grams of zinc oxide are needed to make 120 g of 10% zinc oxide paste?

18. How many grams of boric acid will be needed to make 400 g of a 4% (w/w) ointment?

19. How many grams of strong silver protein (SSP) are required to make 250 ml of a 0.25% (w/v) solution?

20. How many grams of boric acid are there in 1 gallon of a 2% (w/v) boric acid solution?

21. If 10 g of a chemical is dissolved in enough water to make the preparation measure one liter, what is the percentage strength of the solution?

22. How many milliliters of a 0.02% w/v solution can be made from 2.5 g of a chemical?

23. Normal saline solution contains 0.9% w/v NaCl. How many grams of sodium chloride should be used to make 2 liters of normal saline?

Answers

1. 20 ml	2. 12 ml	3. 18 ml
4. 12.5 ml	5. 133 ml	6. 6 ml
7. 100 ml	8. 1260 g	9. 15.3 gallons
10. 31.25 g	11. 3405 g or 7.5lb	12. 0.96 g
13. 200 ml	14. 24 ml	15. 2.4 g
16. 10 g	17. 12	18. 16 g
19. 0.625 g	20. 75.7 g	21. 1%
22. 12,500 ml	23. 18 g	

ALLIGATION METHOD

When the calculation involves mixing of two similar preparations of different strength, to produce a preparation of intermediate strength, the alligation method is used. Alligation is a method used to solve problems that involve mixing two products of different strengths to form a product having a desired intermediate strength. Alligation is used to calculate:

a. The amount of diluent that must be added to a given amount of higher strength preparation to make a desired lower strength.

b. The amounts of active ingredient which must be added to a given amount of lower strength preparation to make a higher strength.

c. The amount of higher and lower strength preparations that must be combined to make a desired amount of an intermediate strength (Figs 1.3A to D).

The method is recommended for the purpose of checking the calculations.

Example: Calculate the volume of 95% alcohol required to prepare 300 ml of 70% alcohol by allegation method?

Calculation:

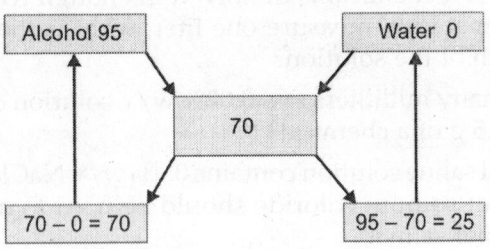

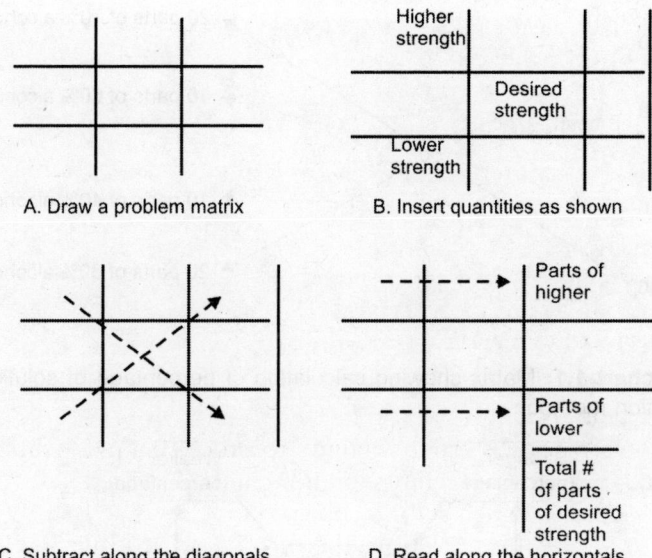

A. Draw a problem matrix

B. Insert quantities as shown

C. Subtract along the diagonals

D. Read along the horizontals

Figs 1.3A to D: Matrix showing percentage calculation method by alligation method

Volume required = 300 ml, percentage of alcohol required = 70, percentage of alcohol used = 95

Using alligation method

70 parts of 95% alcohol and 25 parts of water will produce the required percentage alcohol.

Quantity of 95% alcohol required $= \dfrac{300 \times 70}{95} = 221$ ml

Quantity of water required $= \dfrac{300 \times 25}{9} = 79$ ml.

Hence to produce 300 ml of 70% alcohol, 221 ml of 95% alcohol is to be taken.

Example: Calculate the amount of 70, 60, 40 and 30% alcohol should be mixed to get 50% alcohol.

Calculation

Using alligation method

Hence, when 20 parts of 70% alcohol, 10 parts of 60% alcohol, 10 parts of 40% alcohol and 20 parts of 30% alcohol are mixed together, the resulting solution will produce 50% alcohol.

Pharmaceutics II

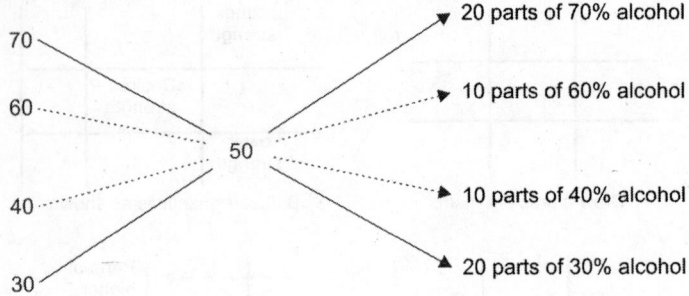

Flowchart 1.1: Matrix showing calculation of percentage of solution by alligation method

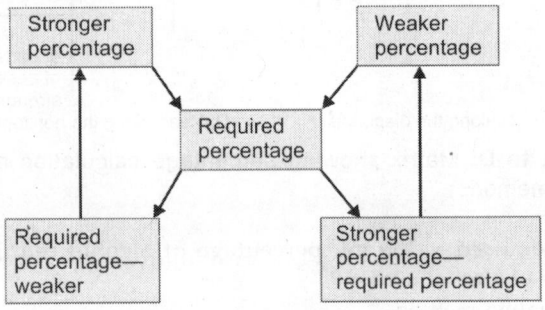

PRACTICE QUESTIONS

1. In what proportion a solution containing 15% of a drug be mixed with 30% of same drug to get 20% mixture concentration?

2. What will be the % of alcohol obtained by mixing a solution containing 5 L of 25%, 1 L of 50% and 2 L of 95% alcohol?

3. In what proportion a solution containing 70% of a drug be mixed with 40% of same drug to get 50% mixture concentration?

4. In what proportion a solution containing 80, 60, 40, and 30% of a drug be mixed with to get 50% mixture concentration?

5. How much water is to be added to 700 ml of 92%, 850 ml of 86% and 600 ml of 26% alcohol to obtain a mixture of 20% strength?

Answers

1. 5 parts of 30% and 10 parts of 15%   2. 45.6%
3. 10 parts of 70% and 20 parts of 40%.   4. 10:20:30:10
5. 5504 ml.

PROOF SPIRIT

For excise purpose, the strength of alcoholic preparations are indicated by degrees, **"over proof"** or **"under proof"**. Proof spirit is that mixture of alcohol and water which at 51°F weighs 12/13th of an equal volume of water.

In India, 57.1 volume of ethyl alcohol is considered to be equal to 100 volumes of proof spirit. This means that any alcoholic solution which contains 57.1% v/v alcohol is a proof spirit which is said to be 100 proof. Hence strength above proof strength is expressed as over proof (OP) and any strength below proof strength is expressed as under proof (UP)

For excise purpose in India the proof alcohol is calculated in terms of rupees per litre of proof alcohol. So any percentage volume in volume of alcohol can be converted into proof strength and vice versa by using the following method:

1. Multiply the percentage strength of alcohol by 1.753 and subtracting 100 from it.
2. If the result is positive, it is known as over proof (OP)
3. If the result is negative, it is known as under proof (UP).

The value 1.753 used in the formula is calculated as

57.1 volumes of ethyl alcohol = 100 volume of proof spirit

1 volume of ethyl alcohol = 100/57.1 = 1.753 volume of proof spirit.

Example: Find strength of 85% v/v alcohol in terms of proof spirit.
Solution:
By applying the formula
Percentage strength of alcohol × 1.73 – 100
$$= 85 \times 1.753 - 100$$
$$= 149 - 100 = + 49, \text{ i.e. } 49° \text{ OP.}$$

Example: Find strength of 60% v/v alcohol in terms of proof spirit.
Solution: By applying the formula

Percentage strength of alcohol × 1.753 – 100
$$= 60 × 1.753–100$$
$$= 105.2–100 = +5.2, \text{ i.e. } 5.2° \text{ OP}$$

Example: Find strength of 45% v/v alcohol in terms of proof spirit.

Solution: By applying the formula
Percentage strength of alcohol × 1.753 – 100
$$= 45 × 1.753 – 100$$
$$= 78.9 – 100 = –21.1, \text{ i.e. } 21.1° \text{ UP}$$

Example: Calculate the strength of 30° OP and 40° UP.

Solution: By applying the formula
30° over proof means 100 + 30 = 130
Alcohol strength = 130/1.753 = 74.15% v/v
(i.e. 74.15% solution diluted to 100 ml qs will give 30° OP solution.)
40° under proof means 100–40 = 60
Alcohol strength = 60/1.753 = 34.23% v/v
(i.e. 34.23% solution diluted to 100 ml qs will give 40° UP solution.)

Example: How many proof gallons are there in 5 of 65% v/v alcohol.

Calculation: Applying the formula
Value in proof = % strength of alcohol × 1.753 – 100
$$= 65 × 1.753 –100$$
$$= 113.9 – 100$$
$$= +13.9$$
$$= 13.9° \text{ OP.}$$

It means
100 gallons of 65% v/v alcohol = 113.9 units of proof spirit
1 gallon of 65% v/v alcohol = 113.9/100

Hence 5 gallons of 65% v/v alcohol $= \dfrac{113.9 × 5}{100}$

$$= 5.7 \text{ gallons of proof spirit}$$

Hence 5 gallons of 65% v/v alcohol are alcohols are equivalent to 5.7 gallons of proof spirit.

PRACTICE QUESTIONS

1. Convert the following degrees of proof into percentage Under proof

   a. 12.1° UP   b. 21.5° UP   c. 54.8° UP

2. Convert the following degrees of proof into percentage over proof

   a. 44.6° OP   b. 35.3° OP   c. 18.4° OP

3. How many proof gallons are therein 5 of 70% v/v alcohol.

Answers

1. a. 50.14%   b. 44.78%   c. 25.78%

2. a. 82.49%   b. 77.18%   c. 67.54%

3. 6.13 gallon

ISOTONIC SOLUTIONS

Solution having the same osmotic pressure is called iso-osmotic. Osmosis is the movement of solvent through a membrane to equalize the concentration on both sides. The pressure required to allow for no transport of solvent across the membrane is called the osmotic pressure and obeys the relation:

$$\pi = \frac{n_{solute}}{V_{soln}} \, RT = MRT$$

Isotonicity: If the concentrations of electrolytes are the same in the cell and surrounding fluid, the situation is balanced (homeostatic). The cell fluid volume remains the same (Fig. 1.4).

Hypertonicity: The cell will shrink (crenation) by loss of its fluid to the surrounding hypertonic environment. High osmotic pressure of surrounding fluid pulls fluid out of the cell (Fig. 1.5).

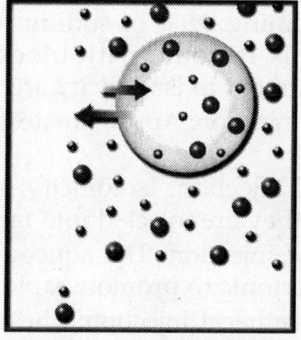

Fig 1.4: Isotonic solution

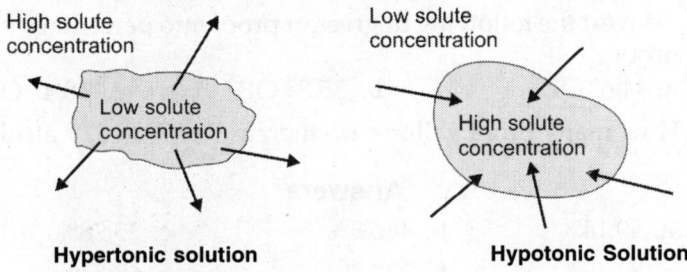

Fig. 1.5: Hypertonic and hypotonic solution

Hypotonicity: In a hypotonic environment, fluid will enter a cell and cause it to swell and burst. The inside of the cell has higher osmotic pressure than the surrounding fluid, so fluid is drawn into the cell.

Both hypertonicity and hypotonicity in the extracellular fluids will destroy cells. Need isotonicity for cell homeostasis, for balance. To determine whether or not a solution is isotonic with erythrocytes, it is necessary to determine the concentration of the solute at which the cells retain their normal size and shape. The parenteral solution and ophthalmic solutions need adjustment to iso-osmoticity and isotonicity.

The solutions which are not having the same osmotic pressure are called 'Paratonic'. Which comparing a solution with the one of known osmotic pressure those which comparing a solution with the one of known osmotic pressure, those which exert a greater pressure are called 'Hypertonic'. Blood make the contains 0.88% of inorganic salts, mainly sodium chloride, which make the main contribution to osmotic pressure.

A solution containing 0.9% of sodium chloride and 5.4% dextrose solution is isotonic with blood plasma general principles for adjustment to isotonicity are:

i. Solutions for IV injection: Approximate isotonicity is always desirable.

ii. Solution for SC injection: Isotonicity is required but not essential since, they are injected into fatty tissues.

iii. Solutions for IM injection: The aqueous solutions should be slightly hypertonic to promote rapid absorption.

iv. Solution for intrathecal injection: These must be isotonic, because the volume of CSF is only 60 to 80 ml. Hence, a small volume of a paratonic solution will disturb the osmotic pressure may cause vomiting and other side effects.

v. Solution used for nasal drops: Isotonicity is needed, since paratonic solution may cause irritation.

vi. Solution used as eyedrops and eye lotion: Eye lotion should be isotonic with lacrimal secretion, since a large volume is brought in with the eye. For washing the eyes hypertonic solutions are used because they causes excessive tear production which helps in draining out of dirty materials from the eye.

Calculation Based on Isotonicity

1. Based on freezing point method

   Percentage w/v of adjusting substance needed = 0.52–a/b

   here, a = Freezing point of the unadjusted solution

   b = Freezing point of a 1% w/v of adjusting substance.

2. Based on molecular concentration

   Percentage w/v of adjusting substance required = 0.03 M/N

Example: Calculate the amount of procaine hydrochloride which will give a solution iso-osmotic with blood plasma? (The freezing point of 1% w/v solution of procaine hydrochloride is –0.122°C).

Calculation: By applying the formula

Percentage w/v of adjusting substance needed = 0.52–a/b

$$= \frac{0.52 - 0.0}{0.122}$$

$$= 4.2\% \text{ w/v}$$

Note: a = 0 (Freezing point of unadjusted solution is to be taken zero when not given).

Example: Calculate the amount of sodium chloride required to make 1% solution of boric acid iso-osmotic with blood plasma? (The freezing point of 1% w/v solution of boric acid is –0.288°C and the freezing point of 1% w/v solution of sodium chloride is –0.576°C).

Calculation: By applying the formula

Percentage w/v of adjusting substance needed = 0.52–a/b

$$= \frac{0.52 - 0.288}{0.576}$$

$$= 0.39\% \ w/v$$

Example: Calculate the amount of sodium chloride required to make 1.5% solution of boric acid iso-osmotic with blood plasma? (The freezing point of 1% w/v solution of boric acid is –0.288°C and the freezing point of 1% w/v solution of sodium chloride is –0.576°C).

Calculation: By applying the formula

Percentage w/v of adjusting substance needed = 0.52–a/b

$$= \frac{0.52 - (0.288 \times 1.5)}{0.576}$$

$$= 0.15\% \ w/v$$

PRACTICE QUESTIONS

1. What concentration of cocaine hydrochloride will give solution iso-osmotic with blood
   Plasma? The freezing point of 1% w/v solution of cocaine hydrochloride is –0.09°C?

2. What concentration of lignocaine hydrochloride will give solution iso-osmotic with blood plasma? The freezing point of 1% w/v solution of cocaine hydrochloride is –0.09°C?

3. What concentration of sodium chloride is required to make 1% solution of adrenaline iso-osmotic with blood plasma? The freezing point of 1% w/v solution of adrenaline is –0.09°C and the freezing point of 1% w/v solution of sodium chloride is –0.576°C?

4. What concentration of sodium chloride is required to make 1.5% solution of procaine hydrochloride iso-osmotic with blood plasma? The freezing point of 1% w/v solution of procaine hydrochloride is –0.122°C and the freezing point of 1% w/v solution of sodium chloride is –0.576°C?

Answers

1. 5.77% w/v   2. 5.71% w/v

3. 0.732% w/v   4. 0.585% w/v

ISOLATED KEY POINTS

- "A medical prescription is an order (often in written form) by a qualified health care professional to a pharmacist or other therapist for a treatment to be provided to their patient".
- R_x symbol similarity to the eye of Horus, others to the ancient symbol for Jupiter, alternatively, it may be intended as an abbreviation of the latin "recipe", the imperative form of "recipere", "to take".
- Parts of a prescription are **Physician (prescriber) information like** (i) doctor's name, designation and registration number, (ii) address with phone number and e-mail, (iii) date of issue of prescription, (iv) prescription number, (required when calling the pharmacy for a refill or for medical claim purposes).
- **Patient information** the name, address, age and sex of the patient help in identifying the prescription.
- The superscription which consists of the heading where the symbol R_x (an abbreviation for recipe, the latin for 'take thou' or 'you take' is found.
- The inscription (body of prescription) comprises an important part of prescription containing- name(s) of drug(s) and their quantities, (ii) other chief ingredients of the prescription with quantity, (iii) instruction regarding dosage form like tablet, capsule, suspension, mixture, etc. and (iv) dose and quantity of prescription.
- The subscription gives specific directions for the pharmacist on how to compound the medication.
- The signatura which gives instructions to the patient. These instructions are preceded by abbreviation 'sig.' from the latin, meaning 'mark.'
- **Renewal gives** the number of times a prescription is to be repeated, is written by the physician under renewal instructions.
- **Signature** finally, the prescription must bear the signature of the prescriber to impart it the legal validity.
- Procedure should be adopted by the pharmacist while handling the prescription for compounding and dispensing are receiving, reading and checking, collecting and weighing the materials, compounding, labeling and packaging.

- Sources of error in prescription are abbreviation, name of the drug, strength of the preparation, dosage form of the drug prescribed, dose, instructions for the patient, incompatibilities.

PRACTICE QUESTIONS
LONG ANSWER TYPE QUESTIONS

1. What is a medical prescription? What are its various parts?
2. Discuss in brief about various part of a prescription? Make a prescription showing its various parts.
3. Enumerate the various steps involved in handling of prescription.
4. How modern method of prescription is different from old method? What are the advantages and disadvantages of modern method of prescription?
5. What care is to be taken in writing a prescription?
6. What are the various sources of error in writing a prescription?
7. Enumerate the various points which is to be considered in mind for writing a good prescription?

OBJECTIVE TYPE QUESTIONS

i. The term R_x is an abbreviation of Latin term which means..........

ii. The term prescription means .... a drug can be prepared.

iii. ....is the main part of prescription which contains the name and quantities of prescribed drugs.

iv. Direction for administration of drug to patient comes under....................

v. The colour used for labeling "For external use only" is ....

vi. Write the Latin term and meaning of following abbreviation.

Latin	Meaning
a. ac	
b. Alt.h.	

c. Aq
d. bis
e. bid
f. bol
g. cc
h. emuls.
i. hr
j. h.s.
k. liq
l. nebul
m. pc
n. p.o.
o. sos
p. tid
q. Ung.

vii. Match the following.

Parts of prescription	Significance
1. Date	A. You take
2. Superscription	B. Help in misses of prescription
3. Inscription	C. Direction to patient
4. Signature	D. Name and quantity of medicine

viii. Match the following

Latin term	Meaning
1. Ad	A. Right ear
2. A	B. To make
3. Fiat	C. Mix
4. Mistura	D. Up to
5. Mitte	E. Send

ix. Superscription contains:
a. Symbol R_x
b. Names and quantities of prescribed ingredients
c. Instruction to the pharmacist
d. Direction to the patient

x. Inscription contains:
a. Symbol R_x
b. Direction to the patient

    c. Names and quantities of prescribed ingredients

    d. Instruction to the pharmacist.

xi. Modern method of prescribing does not include:

    a. handover the ready-made preparations to the patients

    b. To advice regarding its mode of administration.

    c. The practice of writing long, complicated prescriptions containing several ingredients.

    d. To advice regarding the quantity of the drug to be taken.

xii. Medicines which are used externally must be labeled "For external use only" in:

    a. Red or against a red background

    b. Green or against a green background

    c. Black or against a black background

    d. Yellow or against a yellow background

xiii. Prescription abbreviation used for water is:

    a. aq   b. aa

    c. aa   d. ad

xiv. Prescription abbreviation h.s.:

    a. At bedtime

    b. Hour

    c. Hypodermic

    d. None of above

xv. Latin word 'cibos' means:

    a. Food   b. With food

    c. After food   d. Before food

Answers

   i. Recipe (You take)   ii. to write before

 iii. Inscription   iv. Signatura.

  v. Red.   vii. 1. A, 2. A, 3. D, 4. C

viii. 1. D, 2. A, 3. B, 4. C, 5. E   ix. a.

  x. c   xi. c

 xii. c   xiii. a

 xiv. a   xv. a

Chapter 2

Pharmaceutical Incompatibilities

The prescriptions are generally written for the official and proprietary medicines, which are manufactured by the pharmaceutical industries. The prescriptions are rarely compounded and dispensed in these days in chemist's shop or hospital pharmacy.

"Incompatibility occurs as a result of the mixing of two or more antagonistic substance and an undesirable product is formed which may affect the safety, efficacy and appearance of the pharmaceutical preparation". Incompatibility may occur not only during compounding and dispensing but also at any stage during formulation, manufacturing, packaging or administration of drugs.

Types of Incompatibilities

The incompatibilities are of three types

1. Physical incompatibility
2. Chemical incompatibility
3. Therapeutic incompatibility

PHYSICAL INCOMPATIBILITY

Physical incompatibility is usually due to immiscibility, insolubility, precipitate formation or liquefaction of solid materials. The physical incompatibilities may be corrected by using any one or more of the following methods:

1. Immiscibility
2. Insolubility
3. Liquefaction

Immiscibility

a. Oils are immiscible with water and hence combination of oily drugs with water produces a product possessing two separate layers.

   Remedy: This problem can be overcome by emulsification or solubilization.

b. Care must be taken when concentrated hydroalcoholic solutions of volatile oils, such as spirits and concentrated waters, are used as adjuncts (e.g. as flavouring agents) in aqueous preparations. Large globules of oils may be separated.

   Remedy: To prevent the formation of large globules, the hydroalcoholic solution should either be gradually diluted with the vehicle before admixture with the remaining ingredients or poured into the vehicle with constant stirring.

Insolubility

a. Some insoluble powders, such as sulphur and certain corticosteroids (hydrocortisone acetate) and antibiotics are difficult to wet with water.

   Remedy: Wetting agents like saponins for sulphur containing lotions and polysorbates in parenteral suspensions of corticosteroids

b. When a resinous tincture is added to water the water insoluble resin agglomerate forming indiffusible clots.

   Remedy: This is prevented by slowly adding the undiluted dispersion of protective colloid (Tragacanth mucilage), e.g. Lobelia and Stramonium tincture which should be mixed with tragacanth mucilage and stirred constantly. This will produce a stable preparation.

Liquefaction

When certain low melting point solids are powdered together a liquid or soft mass is produced due to lowering of the melting point of the mixture to below room temperature. Thus an eutectic mixture is formed. Any two of the following exhibits this type of behaviour, camphor, menthol, phenol, thymol and chloral hydrate, also sodium salicylate with phenazone, e.g.

R$_x$

Thymol	250 mg
Camphor	2 mg
Menthol	2 mg

Make powder.

Comments: If these ingredients are triturated together, they will form an eutectic mixture.

Method I: All the ingredients are triturated. An eutectic mixture (liquid) will be formed. The liquid is triturated with enough absorbent powder, e.g. light kaolin or light magnesium carbonate, to give a free flowing powder.

Method II: Each ingredient is triturated separately with small amount of adsorbent or diluent and then these powders are lightly mixed by tumbling action and packed. The diluent largely prevents contact between the ingredients and adsorbs any liquid that may be produced, e.g.

R$_x$

Chloral hydrate   250 mg

Prepare capsules. Supply 10 capsules.

Label: Take the capsules at night time.

Comment: Chloral hydrate is hygroscopic in nature. It will absorb moisture and soften the hard gelatin capsule shells and the shape of the capsule may change physically.

Remedy: An equal quantity of light magnesium oxide should be mixed with chloral hydrate. Other adsorbents those may be used are kaolin, talc, starch, etc.

CHEMICAL INCOMPATIBILITY

Chemical incompatibility is due to chemical reactions between the ingredients and a toxic or inactive product may be formed. While dispensing such preparations, precautions should be taken either to prevent the formation of harmful product. Chemical incompatibilities is due to oxidation-reduction, acid base hydrolysis or combination reactions. These reactions leads to precipitation, effervescence, decomposition, colour change or by explosion.

Chemical incompatibilities are of two types:

1. **Tolerated:** In tolerated incompatibilities, the chemical interaction are minimized by changing the order of mixing or mixing the solutions in dilute forms.

2. **Adjusted:** In adjusted incompatibilities the chemical interaction are prevented by addition or substitution of one of the reacting ingredients of a prescription with another of equal therapeutic value.

The chemical incompatibility may be: (i) Intentional: When the prescriber knowingly prescribes the incompatible drugs; (ii) Unintentional: When the prescriber prescribes the drugs without knowing that there is incompatibility between the prescribed drugs.

Examples of Chemical Incompatibilities
Alkaloidal Incompatibility

i. **Alkaloidal salts with alkaline substances:** Alkaloids are weak bases. They are almost insoluble in water but alkaloidal salts are soluble in water. If these salts are dispensed with alkaline preparations, such as strong solution of ammonium acetate, aromatic spirit of ammonia, solution of ammonia, ammonium bicarbonate, sodium bicarbonate, the free alkaloid may be precipitated, e.g.

R_x

Strychnine hydrochloride solution	6 ml
Ammonium acetate	4 ml
Water up to	120 ml

Make a mixture.

Strychnine hydrochloride is an alkaloidal salt while ammonium acetate is an alkaline substance. When they react together, the strychnine gets precipitated because the quantity of strychnine hydrochloride prescribed in the prescription is much more than its solubility in water. The ammonium acetate contains negligible amount of alcohol which cannot dissolve the strychnine. Hence, it gets precipitated as diffusible precipitate. Hence follow method A for precipitate yielding combination.

ii. **Alkaloidal salts with salicylates:** When quinine compounds are combined with salicylates, it forms indiffusible precipitates of quinine salicylate, e.g.

Quinine hydrochloride	0.12 g
Sodium salicylate	4.0 g
Water q.s	100 ml

Quinine hydrochloride on reaction with sodium salicylate forms quinine salicylate which gets separated as indiffusible precipitate.

Soluble Salicylates Incompatibilities

i. **Soluble salicylates with ferric salt:** Ferric salf reacts with sodium salicylate to liberate indiffusible precipitates of ferric salicylate, e.g.

Ferric chloride solution	0.2 ml
Sodium salicylate	0. 3 g
Water up to	9 ml

Make a mixture.

Ferric chloride reacts with sodium salicylate to form ferric salicylate which gets separated as indiffusible precipitate.

Chemical Incompatibilities Causing Evolution of Carbon Dioxide Gas

When carbonates or bicarbonates comes in contact of an acid or acidic drug in a mixture, they react together with the evolution of carbon dioxide gas. If the reaction is not allowed to complete before transferring the mixture into a dispensing bottle and corked, there are chances of explosion with bursting of the bottle. To prevent explosion, the reaction must be completed before dispensing the mixture. To speed up the reaction mixed the ingredients in an open vessel and allow the reaction to complete until effervescence ceases.

THERAPEUTIC INCOMPATIBILITY

Usually, this incompatibility arises when one or more drugs produces response or intensity different from that intended in the patients. It may be due to following below mentioned reasons:

1. Overdose
2. Underdose
3. Contraindicated drugs
4. Drug interactions

Overdose

Excessive single dose: Sometimes a single dose may become overdose depending on the health of the patient, e.g. a normal dose (taking body weight as 70 kg as standard for an adult male) may be overdose for a underweight person, e.g.

R_x
Atropine sulphate   6 mg
Phenobarbital   360 mg
Make capsules.

Label: One capsule to be taken three times a day before meals.

Remedy: In this prescription the doses of both atropine sulphate and phenobarbital are 12 times the normal doses. The physician intended for 12 capsules to be dispensed but he has mistaken or may be it is an incomplete prescription. Hence, before dispensing the pharmacist should consult the physician again.

Correct prescription

R_x
Atropine sulphate   6 mg
Phenobarbital   360 mg
Make capsules. Supply 12 capsules.

Label: One capsule to be taken three times a day before meals, e.g.

R_x
Strychnine sulphate   20 mg
Iron and ammonium citrate   500 mg
Prepare capsules. Supply 12 capsules.

Label: One capsule to be taken three times a day after meals.

Comment: 10 times overdose of strychnine hydrochloride than that of normal. The pharmacist should consult the physician and obtain the permission to change the dose.

Corrected prescription

Strychnine sulphate	2 mg
Iron and ammonium citrate	500 mg

Prepare capsules. Supply 12 capsules.

Label: One capsule to be taken three times a day after meals.

Excessive daily dose: In this case the daily dose of drug is exceeded, e.g.

R_x

Codeine phosphate	15 mg
Ammonium chloride	500 mg

Prepare capsules and supply 24 capsules.

Label: Two capsules to be taken every hour for cough.

Remedy: As per The USP the prescribed dose should be taken after every four hours and not every hour. Hence, the physician should be consulted.

Additive and synergistic combinations: There are certain drugs possessing similar pharmacological activity. If these drugs are combined together, they may produce additive or synergistic action. Hence, the physician should be consulted, e.g.

R_x

Amphetamine sulphate	20 mg
Ephedrine sulphate	50 mg
Syrup q.s.	100 ml

Make a mixture

Label: Take 25 ml every four hours.

Remedy: Both of the drugs have synergistic effect. The formulation will produce overdose effect. Hence, the dose of individual drug should be reduced.

Underdose

In this type of incompatibility, effect of one drug is lessen or antagonised by the presence of another drug. This can be exemplified by combination of following types of drugs:

1. Stimulants like nux vomica, caffeine, etc. with sedatives like barbiturates, paraldehyde, etc.
2. Purgatives like castor oil, liquid paraffin, etc. with antidiarrheal agents like bismuth carbonates.
5. Acidifiers like dilute hydrochloric acid and alkalisers like sodium bicarbonate, magnesium carbonate, e.g.

R_x

Aspirin	300 mg
Probenecid	500 mg

Prepare capsules.

Label: One capsule a day for gout.

Aspirin is an NSAID given to reduce the pain and swelling in case of gout attack. Probenecid blocks the active reabsorption of uric acid from the lumen of nephron, but salicylates (aspirin) blocks this action of probenecid. Hence, both of the drugs are antagonistic to each other, so its combination is therapeutically useless.

Contraindicated Drugs

Certain drugs should not be given in particular disease condition, e.g.

i. Corticosteroids are contraindicated in patients with peptic ulcer.
ii. Vasoconstrictors are contraindicated in hypertensive patients
iii. Certain combination of drugs are contraindicate, e.g.

R_x

Sulphadiazine	0.25 g
Sulphamerazine	0.25 g
Ammonium chloride	0.50 g

Prepare capsules

Label: Take two capsules six hourly for cough.

Comment: In this prescription ammonium chloride is a urinary acidifier and it could cause deposition of sulphonamide crystals in the kidney.

Drug Interactions

The effect of one drug is altered by the prior or simultaneous administration of another drug. The drug interactions can usually be corrected by the proper adjustment of dosage if the suspected interaction is detected, e.g.

Acetophenetidin	150 mg
Acetyl salicylic acid	200 mg
Caffeine	30 mg

Send ten capsules.

Acetophenetidin and acetyl salicylic acid are analgesics. Acetophenetidin depresses the CNS and this side effect is undesirable. Caffeine is a CNS stimulant to neutralize the side effect of acetophenetidin. The incompatibility is intentional, e.g.

R_x

Tetracycline hydrochloride 250 mg

Prepare capsules. Supply 10 capsules.

Label: Take one capsule every six hourly.

Comments: Calcium present in milk inactivates the tetracycline, hence a patient may not get any therapeutic effect if he/she takes the capsule with milk.

Remedy: The pharmacist should advise the patient to take the capsule with water and not with milk. The patient should not take antacid containing calcium salts.

ISOLATED KEY POINTS

- Incompatibility occurs as a result of the mixing of two or more antagonistic substance and an undesirable product is formed which may affect the safety, efficacy and appearance of the pharmaceutical preparation.
- There are three types of incompatibilities physical incompatibility, chemical incompatibility, therapeutic incompatibility.
- Physical incompatibility occur when two or more than two substances are mixed together, a physical change takes place and an unacceptable product is formed.

- Physical incompatibility is usually due to immiscibility, insolubility, precipitate formation or liquefaction of solid materials.
- Chemical incompatibility is due to chemical reactions between the ingredients and a toxic or inactive product may be formed.
- Chemical incompatibilities is due to oxidation-reduction, acid base hydrolysis or combination reactions. These reactions leads to precipitation, effervescence, decomposition, colour change or by explosion.
- Chemical incompatibilities are of two types:
  - a. Tolerated: In tolerated incompatibilities, the chemical interaction are minimized by changing the order of mixing or mixing the solutions in dilute forms.
  - b. Adjusted: In adjusted incompatibilities, the chemical interaction are prevented by addition or substitution of one of the reacting ingredients of a prescription with another of equal therapeutic value.
- Therapeutic incompatibility arises when one or more drugs produces response or intensity different from that intended in the patients.
- Therapeutic incompatibility is due to following reasons, overdoses, underdoses, contraindicated drugs, drug interactions.

PRACTICE QUESTIONS
LONG ANSWER TYPE QUESTIONS

1. What are the various types of incompatibilities in prescription? Discuss in brief.
2. What is physical incompatibility? How it occurs, give examples?
3. What is chemical incompatibility? Differentiate between tolerated and adjusted chemical incompatibility?
4. What is alkaloidal incompatibility? Give some examples.
5. How chemical incompatibility occur which involves evolution of carbon dioxide gas?
6. What is therapeutic incompatibility? Discuss in brief about the various reasons due to which therapeutic incompatibility occurs?

OBJECTIVE TYPE QUESTIONS

i. Match the following:

Compatibility	Cause
1. Physical	A. Error in writing
2. Chemical	B. Immiscibility
3. Therapeutic	C. Oxidation-reduction

ii. Medicines which are used externally must be labeled "For external use only" in:
   a. Red or against a red background
   b. Green or against a green background
   c. Black or against a block background
   d. Yellow or against a yellow background

iii. Physical incompatibility may not occur due to:
   a. Immiscibility
   b. Insolubility
   c. Precipitate formation
   d. Oxidation

iv. In .... compatibility the chemical interaction are minimized by changing the order of mixing or mixing the solutions in dilute forms:
   a. Tolerated   b. Adjusted
   c. Intentional   c. Unintentional

Answers

i. 1. B, 2. C, 3. A   ii. a

iii. d   iv. a

Chapter 3

Posology

The term posology is derived from Greek word '**Poso**' meaning *"how much"* and '**Logos**' meaning *"science"*. Hence posology is a branch which deals with dose or quantity of drugs which can be administered to a patient to get desired pharmacological and therapeutic action. The dose cannot be fixed rigidly because there are so many factors which influence the doses. These factors are age, condition of the patient, severity of disease, tolerances both natural and acquired, idiosyncrasy, route of administration, type of formulation, drug interaction and rate of excretion.

Factors Affecting Dose

The optimum dose of a drug which produces the desired therapeutic effect varies from person to person, the dose range is usually based on the average requirement of an adult person depending upon his body weight, height, surface area and other parameters. The following are some factor which affect the dose:

Age: The pharmacokinetics **(ADME)** of many drugs changes with age. Hence while determining the dose of a drug, the age of an individual is of great importance. Children and old people need lesser amount of drug than the normal adult dose, because they are unable to excrete drugs to that extent as adults. In children the various organs are less developed as compared to an adult one, especially in case of neonates special care is to be taken to dispense the drug.

Sex: Women do not always respond to action of drugs in same manner as man. Morphine and barbiturates may produce more excitement before sedation in women. Special care should be taken when drugs are administered during menstruation, pregnancy and lactation. The strong purgatives such as aloes should be avoided during menstruation. Similarly the drugs which may stimulate the uterine smooth muscle, e.g. drastic purgatives, ant—malarial drugs and ergot alkaloids are contraindicated during pregnancy. There are certain drugs which on administration to the mother are capable of crossing the placenta and affecting the fetus, e.g. alcohol, narcotics, barbiturates and non narcotics analgesics, etc. During lactation, the drugs like antihistaminic, morphine and tetracycline which are excreted in milk should be avoided or given very cautiously to the mothers who are breastfeeding the babies.

Body weight: The average dose is mentioned either in terms of mg per kg body weight or as a total single dose for an adult weighing between 50 o 100 kg. The dose expressed in this manner may not apply in case of obese patients, children and malnourished patients. It should be calculated according to body weight.

Route of administration: Intravenous doses of drugs are usually smaller than oral doses, because the drugs administered intravenously reaches the systemic circulation, i.e. the blood stream directly. Due to this reason the onset of drug action is quick with intravenous route and this might enhance the chances of drug toxicity. The effectiveness of drug formulation is generally controlled by the route of administration. For example, the same drug ranitidine can be given orally as well as parenteral route depending upon the type of severity of disease and condition of the patient.

Time of administration: The presence of food in the stomach delays absorption of drugs. The drugs are more rapidly absorbed from the empty stomach. So, the amount of drug which is very effective when taken before meal may not be that much effective when taken during or after meals. Antacids are to be given before meals similarly enzymes preparation are to be given after meals.

Patient status: The personality and behaviour of a patient may influence the effect of drug, especially the drug which is more intended for psychosomatic disorders. The females are more emotional than males and require lower dose of certain drugs. Inert dosage forms called placebos which resemble the actual medicament in physical properties are known to produce therapeutic benefit in diseases like angina pectoris and bronchial asthma.

Presence of disease: Drugs like barbiturates and chlorpromazine may produce unusually prolonged effects in patients liver cirrhosis. Streptomycin is excreted mainly by the kidney may prove toxic if the kidney of patient is not working properly. Similarly patient suffering from liver ailment like jaundice than oral route is not preferred, drug is given parenteral so as to by pass liver. During fever a patient can tolerate high doses of antipyretics than a normal person.

Cumulative Effect: The drugs which are slowly excreted may build up a sufficiently high concentration in the body and produce toxic symptoms, if it is repeatedly administered for a long time, e.g. digitalis, emetine and heavy metals. This occurs due to accumulative effect of the drug. The cumulative effects are usually produced by slow excretion, degradation and rapid absorption of drugs. Sometimes, a cumulative effect is desire in drugs like phenobarbitone in treatment of epilepsy.

Additive effect: When the total pharmacological action of two or more drugs administered together is equivalent to sum of their individual; pharmacological action, the phenomena is called an additive effect. For example, combination of paracetamol and ibuprofen for analgesic effect.

Synergism: When two or more drugs used in combination form, their action is more than the individual effect of the drug. The phenomenon is called synergism. Synergism is very useful when desired therapeutic result needed is difficult to achieve with a single drug, e.g. procaine and adrenaline combination, increases the duration of action of procaine.

Idiosyncrasy (Hypersensitivity reaction): An extraordinary response to a drug which is different from its characteristic pharmacological action is called idiosyncrasy. It is also called hypersensitivity reaction. There is difference in the term side effect and word idiosyncrasy, when a person is taking a drug then apart from its pharmacological action the drug is also causing some unwanted effects in the body these are called side effects while if a person is sensitive to a particular drug then on taking that drug allergic reactions takes place which can cause severe toxicity also these are termed idiosyncrasy. Fro example, on taking a tablet of paracetamol some damage will occur to liver this is side effect of drug while if skin rashes appear than it is idiosyncrasy. Some persons are sensitive to penicillin and sulphonamides because they produce severe toxic symptoms.

Tachyphylaxis: It has been observed that when certain drugs are administered repeated at short intervals, the cell receptors get blocked up and pharmacological response to that particular drug is decreased. The decreased response cannot be reversed by increasing the dose. This phenomenon is known as tachyphylaxis or acute tolerance. For example, ephedrine when given in repeated dose at short intervals in treatment of bronchial asthma may produce very less response due to tachyphylaxis.

CALCULATION OF DOSES

The doses of a drug given represent the average maximum quantity of drugs which can be administered to an adult orally within 24 hours. When others routes of administration are followed, the dose is adjusted accordingly. The doses are also calculated in proportion to age, body weight and surface area of the patient.

1. Doses proportionate to age: There are a number of methods by which the dose for a child can be calculated from adult dose.

Young's formula:

$$\text{Dose of a child} = \frac{\text{Age in years}}{\text{Age} + 12} \times \text{Adult dose}$$

The formula is used for calculating the doses of children less than 12 years of age.

Dilling's formula:

$$\text{Dose of a child} = \frac{\text{Age in years}}{20} \times \text{Adult dose}$$

The formula is used for calculating the doses for children in between 4 and 20 years of age. This formula is considered better because it is easier and quick to calculate the dose.

Cowling's Formula:

$$\text{Dose of a child} = \frac{\text{Age at next birthday}}{24} \times \text{Adult dose}$$

Fried's Formula:

$$\text{Dose of a child} = \frac{\text{Age at next months}}{150} \times \text{Adult dose}$$

This formula is most useful for calculating the dose of kids less than 2 years of age.

Bastedo's Formula:

$$\text{Dose of a child} = \frac{\text{Age in years} + 3}{30} \times \text{Adult dose}$$

2. Doses proportionate to body weight: Clark's formula is used to calculate the dose for child according to body weight.

Clark's formula:

$$\text{Dose of a child} = \frac{\text{Weight in pounds}}{150} \times \text{Adult dose}$$

3. Doses proportionate to Surface Area:

$$\text{Dose of a child} = \frac{\text{Body surface area of child}}{\text{Body surface area of adult}} \times \text{Adult dose}$$

The calculation of child dose according to surface area is most satisfactory and appropriate rater than method based on age. The method is more complicated than method based on age. The body surface area is calculated from height and weight of the child. Table 3.1 shows the determination of children doses from adult doses on the basis of body surface area.

Veterinary Prescription

Veterinary prescription drugs are those drugs which are prescribed by a licensed veterinary doctor to animals for their disease or ailments.

Table 3.1: Determination of children's dose from adult dose on the basis of body surface area

Sl. No.	Weight (Kg)	Approx. Surface area in square metres	Approx. Percentage of adult dose
1.	2	0.15	9
2.	4	0.25	14
3.	6	0.33	19
4.	8	0.40	23
5.	10	0.46	27
6.	15	0.63	36
7.	20	0.80	46
8.	25	0.95	55
9.	30	1.08	62
10.	35	1.20	70
11.	40	1.30	75
12.	45	1.40	81
13.	50	1.51	87
14.	55	1.58	91

A written prescription for a veterinary medicine must include the following information (Fig. 3.1).

  i. Name, address, and telephone number of veterinary doctor
 ii. Name, address, and telephone number of person taking care of animal
iii. Identification (including the species) of the animal
 iv. Date of treatment, prescribing, or dispensing of drug (RPL)
  v. Name, active ingredient, and quantity of the drug to be prescribed or dispensed to the animal
 vi. Drug strength
vii. Dosage and duration
viii. Route of administration
 ix. Veterinary doctor qualifications
  x. Premises at which the animals are kept
 xi. Necessary warnings
xii. Signature of the veterinary doctor

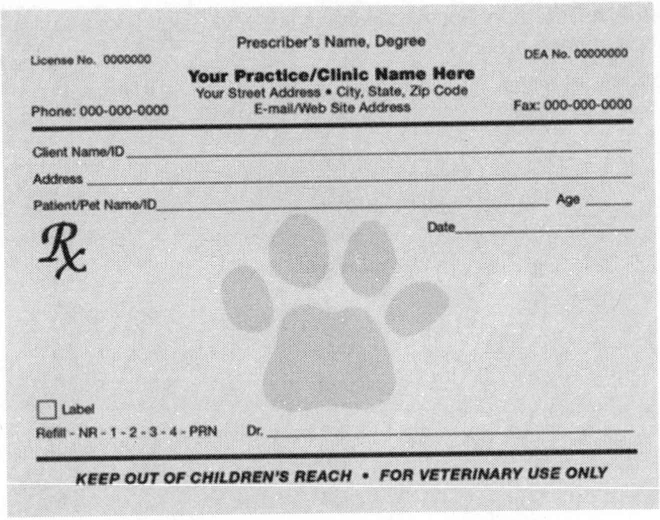

License No. 0000000
Prescriber's Name, Degree
DEA No. 0000000
Your Practice/Clinic Name Here
Your Street Address • City, State, Zip Code
E-mail/Web Site Address
Phone: 000-000-0000
Fax: 000-000-0000

Client Name/ID ____________________
Address ____________________
Patient/Pet Name/ID ____________________ Age ______
Date ____________________

℞

☐ Label
Refill - NR - 1 - 2 - 3 - 4 - PRN Dr. ____________________

KEEP OUT OF CHILDREN'S REACH • FOR VETERINARY USE ONLY

Fig. 3.1: A typical veterinary prescription

Compounding of Veterinary Drugs

Compounding is done by either a veterinarian or by a pharmacist upon the prescription of a veterinarian, to meet the needs of a particular animal. For example, mixing two injectable drugs is compounding. Preparing a paste or suspension from crushed tablets is another example of compounding. Likewise, adding flavouring to a drug is compounding.

i. Compounding must be done by or under the order of a veterinarian.
ii. A compounded human drug cannot be used in a food-producing animal if a legally compounded animal drug can instead be used.
iii. Compounded drugs must be prepared from FDA-approved drugs.
iv. The volume of compounded drug must be in accordance with the need of individual animal.

Handling, Storage and Disposal

Adequate written treatment records must be maintained by the veterinarian for at least two years.

The veterinarian should inform clients to whom prescription drugs are delivered or dispensed about appropriate drug handling, storage, and disposal.

In the clinic, veterinary prescription drugs should be stored separately from over-the-counter drugs, and be easily distinguishable by the professional and paraprofessional staff. Drugs should be stored under conditions recommended by the manufacturer. All drugs should be examined periodically to ensure cleanliness and current dating.

Food animal clients should be advised that veterinary prescription drugs should be securely stored, with access limited to key personnel.

ISOLATED KEY POINTS

- The term posology is derived from greek word 'poso' meaning *"how much"* and 'logos' meaning *"science"*.
- Posology is a branch which deals with dose or quantity of drugs which can be administered to a patient to get desired pharmacological and therapeutic action.
- Factors affecting dose are age, sex, body weight, route of administration, time of administration, patient status, presence of disease, cumulative effect, additive effect, synergism, idiosyncrasy (hypersensitivity reaction), tachyphylaxis.
- Calculation of doses the doses are also calculated in proportion to age, body weight and surface area of the patient.
- **Young's formula:**

$$\text{Dose of a child} = \frac{\text{Age in years}}{\text{Age} + 12} \times \text{Adult dose}$$

- **Dilling's formula:**

$$\text{Dose of a child} = \frac{\text{Age in years}}{20} \times \text{Adult dose}$$

- **Cowling's formula:**

$$\text{Dose of a child} = \frac{\text{Age at next birthday}}{24} \times \text{Adult dose}$$

- **Fried's formula:**

$$\text{Dose of a child} = \frac{\text{Age in months}}{150} \times \text{Adult dose}$$

- **Bastedo's formula:**

$$\text{Dose of a child} = \frac{\text{Age in years} + 3}{30} \times \text{Adult dose}$$

- **Clark's formula:**

$$\text{Dose of a child} = \frac{\text{Weight in pounds}}{150} \times \text{Adult dose}$$

$$\text{Dose of a child} = \frac{\text{Body surface area of child}}{\text{Body surface area of adult}} \times \text{Adult dose}$$

PRACTICE QUESTIONS

1. If the adult dose for a drug is 60 mg, what will be the dose (according to Young's formula) for
   a. 6 years child   b. 8 years child

2. If the adult dose for a drug is 200 mg, what will be the dose (according to Dilling's formula) for
   a. 12 years child   b. 16 years child

3. If the adult dose for a drug is 100 mg, what will be the dose for a
   a. 6 months child   b. 24 months child

4. If the adult dose for a drug is 100 mg, what will be the dose (according to Bastedo's formula) for a
   a. 9 years child   b. 12 years child

5. If the adult dose for a drug is 100 mg, what will be the dose for a child weighing
   a. 24 lbs
   b. 15 lbs

6. If the adult dose for a drug is 60 mg, what will be the dose for a child having surface area 1.2 m^2.

7. The adult dose of a drug is 10 milligrams per kilogram of body weight. How many grams should be given to a patient weighing 220 lbs.?

8. The adult dose of ampicillin suspension is 250 mg/5 ml four times daily. If a child is 3 ft 6 inches tall and weighs 93 lbs., how many milligrams will she receive for each dose?

9. If the usual dose of a drug is 200 milligrams, what would be the dose for an 8-year-old child who weighs 80 lbs.?

Answers

1a. 20 mg   b. 16 mg

2a. 120 mg   b. 160 mg

3a. 4 mg   b. 16 mg

4a. 40 mg   b. 50 mg

5a. 16 mg   b. 10 mg

 6. 41.6 mg   7. 1 g

 8. 166.18 mg or 3 ml

 9. Fried's
    Rule: 128 mg, Young's
    Rule: 80 mg, Clark's
    Rule: 106.6 or 107 mg

Chapter 4

Powders

The solid dosage forms are available mostly in unit dosage forms, (consisting of doses which are taken by numbers) such as tablets, capsules, pills, cachets or powders. When drugs are to be administered orally in dry state, tablets and capsules are the most convenient dosage form. They are effective and patients have no problem in their handling and administration. Some solids are packed and supplied in bulk powder. The bulk powders. The bulk powders meant for external use are dusting powders, insufflations, snuffs and tooth powders. The bulk powders meant for internal use are supplied either as granules or fine powder.

A pharmaceutical powder is a mixture of finely divided drug and/or chemicals in dry form. These are solid dosage form of medicament which are meant for internal and external use. They are available in crystalline or amorphous form. The particle size of powder plays an important role in physical, chemical and biological properties of the dosage forms (Flowchart 4.1). There is a relationship between particle size of powder and dissolution, absorption and therapeutic efficacy of drugs.

Advantages of Powders

i. Powders are one of the oldest dosage form and are used both internally and externally.

ii. Powders are more stable than liquid dosage form.

iii. It is convenient for the physician to prescribe a specific amount of powdered medicament depending upon the need of the patient.

Flowchart 4.1: Showing various solid dosage form

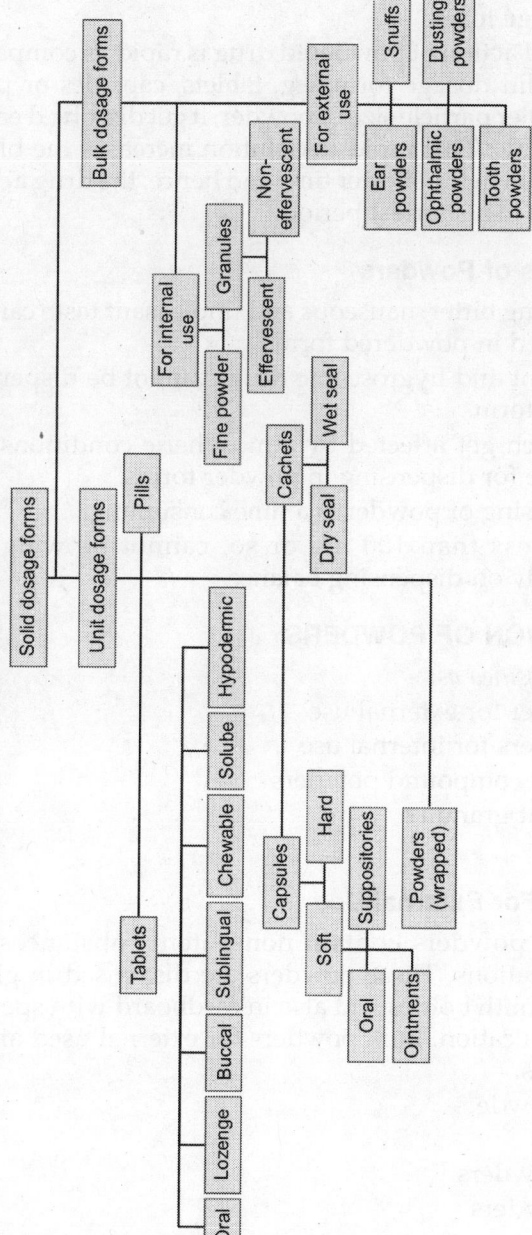

iv. The chances of incompatibility are less as compared to liquid dosage form.

v. The onset of action of powdered drug is rapid as compared to other solid dosage form, e.g. tablets, capsules or pills. Due to smaller particle size of powder, it get dissolved easily in body fluids. This rapid dissolution increases the blood concentration in the shorter time and hence, the drug action is produces in a shortest period.

Disadvantages of Powders

i. Drugs having bitter, nauseous and unpleasant taste cannot be dispensed in powdered form.

ii. Deliquescent and hygroscopic drugs cannot be dispensed in powder form.

iii. Drugs which get affected by atmospheric conditions are not suitable for dispensing in powder forms.

iv. The dispensing of powder is a time consuming.

v. Quantity less than 100 mg or so, cannot be weighed conveniently on dispensing balance.

CLASSIFICATION OF POWDERS

Powders are classified as:
1. Bulk powder for external use
2. Bulk powders for internal use
3. Simple and compound powders
4. Effervescent granules
5. Cachets.

Bulk Powder For External Use

External bulk powders contain non-potent substances for external applications. These powders are dispensed in glass, plastic wide mouth bottles and also in cardboard with specific method of application. Bulk powders for external used are of following types.

a. Dusting powders
b. Snuffs
c. Douche powders
d. Dental powders
e. Insufflation.

Dusting Powders

Dusting powders usually contain substances, such as zinc oxide, starch and boric acid or natural mineral substances, such as kaolin or talc.

Talc may be contaminated with pathogenic microorganisms such as clostridium tetani, etc. and hence, it should be sterilized by dry heat. Dusting powders should not be applied to broken skin. If desired, powders should be micronised or passed through a sieve #80 or 100. Dusting powders should preferably be dispensed in sifter-top containers. Such containers provide the protection from air, moisture and contamination as well as convenience of application. Currently some foot powders and talcum powders have been marketed as pressure aerosols.

Dusting powders are employed chiefly as lubricants, protectives, absorbents, antiseptics, antipruritics, astringents. and antiperspirants.

R_x

Zinc oxide	200 parts
Salicylic acid	20 parts
Starch powder	780 parts(q.s)

Snuffs

These are finely divided solid dosage forms of medicaments dispensed in flat metal boxes with hinged lid. These powders are inhaled into nostrils for decongestion, antiseptic, and bronchodilator action.

Douche Powders

These powders are intended to be used as antiseptics or cleansing agents into the body cavity; most commonly for vaginal use although they may be formulated for nasal, otic or ophthalmic use also. As douche powder formation often include aromatic oils, it becomes necessary to pass them through a # 40 or 60 sieve to eliminate agglomeration and to ensure complete mixing. They can be dispensed either in wide mouth glass bottles or in powder boxes.

R_x

Zinc sulphate	2.5 g
Magnesium sulphate	200 g

Boric acid	30 g
Oil of lemon	0.2 g
Water	1000 ml (qs)

Dental Powders

Dental powders are meant for cleaning the teeth. Dental powders contain detergents, abrasives, antiseptics and colouring and flavouring agents incorporated in a suitable base. Generally, the base is calcium carbonate. The detergent is in the form of soap and finely powdered pumice stone provides abrasive action. Essential oils, if present in small quantity, are easily absorbed by calcium carbonate and pumice. This makes the uniform distribution of the oil difficult.

Insufflation

Insufflations are a class of powders meant for application to body cavities, e.g. ear, nose, vagina, etc. The powder has to be extremely fine and must find an entry to the cavity deep enough to bring about its action at the site. It is delivered to the effected part in a stream with the help of the device called an insufflators, which blow the powder to the site. Some of the insufflations contain volatile liquid ingredients which may require uniform distribution in the powder. Active volatile liquid present in small portion should not be removed by evaporation but only incorporated by trituration in the powder. The pharmaceutical industry packages the insufflations in pressurized form, i.e. aerosols. Aerosols contain the medication in a stout container with a suitable valve, the delivery of the powder being accomplished by a liquefied or compressed gas propellant of a very low boiling point. On pressing the actuator of the valve the propellant delivers the medication in a stream.

Bulk Powder for Internal Use

Bulk powders contain many doses in a wide-mouth container that is suitable to remove the powder by teaspoon. The non-potent substances are used in bulk powder form such an antacids, laxative, purgative, etc.

R_x

| Rhubarb powder | 250 g |
| Light magnesium carbonate | 325 g |

Heavy magnesium carbonates   325 g
Ginger powder   100 g
Make a powder

Simple and Compound Powder for Internal Use

These are unit dose powders normally packed in properly folded papers and dispensed in envelopes, metal foils, small heat-sealed plastic bags or other containers.

Usually for the preparation of simple powders, the ingredients are weighed correctly and blended by geometrical mixing in ascending order of weights. The mixture is then either delivered into blocks of equal size, numbers of blocks representing the number of powder to be dispensed or each dose is weighed separately and placed on a powder paper. The paper is then folded according to the pharmaceutical art and placed in either an envelope or a powder box.

Effervescent Granules

This class of preparation can be supplied either by compounding the ingredients as granules or dispensed in the form of salts. The ingredients whether in granular form represent as salts, react in presence of water evolving carbon dioxide gas. For evolution of the gas two constituents are essential, a soluble carbonate such as sodium bicarbonate and an organic acid such as citric or tartaric acid. The preparation can be supplied either as a bulk powder or distributed in individual powders.

There are three alternative methods of dispensing depending upon the nature of prescription.

If the effervescent salts are prescribed to be the dispensed in bulk form, no granulation is necessary. The ingredients are mixed uniformly and directions stated on the label to add the prescribed quantity to water, before use.

1. If the effervescent salt is prescribed in divided doses, the ingredients, which cause effervescence on mixing with water, are enclosed separately in papers of different colour and add to the water, before use. Quantities of the sodium bicarbonate and the organic acid, citric or tartaric, are in equimolecular in proportion.

2. In the third case the product contains all the ingredients mixed together in a granular form. Preparation of granular

products requires pharmaceutical technique. If sodium bicarbonate and citric acid are taken in equimolecular proportion and mixed to make granules, the quantity of water of crystallization liberated from the citric acid is large enough to make the mass wet and carbon dioxide may be liberated during the preparation itself. If one tries to substitute citric acid by tartaric acid, which contains no water of crystallization; it may not be possible to form a mass necessary to granulation. Therefore both citric and tartaric acid are taken in suitable proportion leaving a little acid in surplus than the quantity required to neutralize sodium bicarbonate. This surplus is necessary to give the final preparation an acidic taste that is more palatable. There is a certain loss in weight of such a preparation due to loss of water in drying the granules and partial loss of carbon dioxide due to its release during preparation. Heating is done on a water bath keeping all the ingredients mixed in a porcelain dish. Gentle application of heat liberates the water of crystallization from citric acid and the mass tends to be coherent. The coherent mass is transferred from the porcelain dish and the granules are dried in an oven taking care to regulate the temperature which should be generally kept below 253 K. If necessary, the dry granules are passed through a sieve of appropriate size to break larger granules, which result due to sticking of the sieved wet granules.

Cachets

Cachet as a unit dosage form was very popular sometime back. Presently cachets are seldom used and have been replaced by capsules. Cachets, like capsules, can be easily filled and sealed at the dispensing counter. This dosage form holds larger quantity of the medication as compared to capsules. Since, the cachets are made of flour and water they are easily damaged in handling. Further this dosage form offers little protection against light and moisture. Due to its size and shape a cachet is difficult to swallow. The process of filling is similar to that of capsules. The drug is placed in one of the two halves of the cachets; the upper half is then placed over it and pressed with the help of a suitable device.

WEIGHING METHODS

Weighing scales (or **weigh scales** or **scales**) are devices to measure weight. **Spring balances** or **spring scales** calculate weight that is the product of mass into gravity (9.807 m/s^2) on the force on a spring, whereas a balance or pair of scales using a balance beam compares masses by balancing the weight due to the mass of an object against the weight of one or more known masses.

Balances Used for Pharmacy

Pharmacy are a well-developed industrial branch, which utilized broad range of balances. For the purpose of warehouse management, four load cell scales are used. Such scales are also used for distribution of big loads into smaller ones. Production stage utilizes single load cell scales, precision and analytical balances. Laboratory tests are based on analytical balances, semi-microbalances and microbalances (ultra-microbalances). The names to above mentioned balances are given according to below relations (Table 4.1).

WEIGHING TECHNIQUES

1. **Top loader:** It is of two types
   A. Direct
   B. Indirect

Direct Weighing

   i. With nothing on the pan, set to zero by pressing the "on" button (Fig. 4.1).
   ii. Place weighing bottle, beaker, or vial on balance and set to zero again.

Table 4.1: Various types of balances and their resolution

S.No	Balance name	Resolution	Quantity of decimal digits
1	Ultra-microbalances	0.1 µg	0.0000001
2	Microbalances	1 µg	0.000001
3	Semi-microbalances	0.01 mg	0.00001
4	Analytical balances	0.1 mg	0.0001

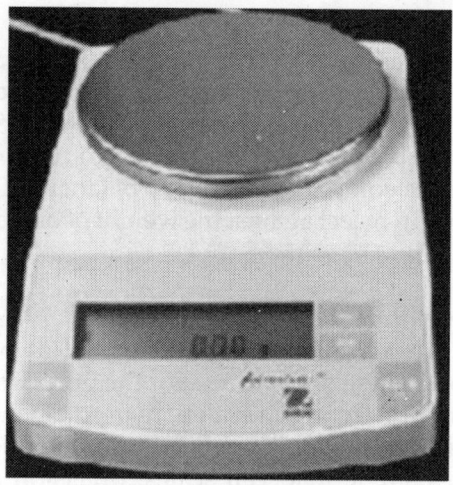

Fig. 4.1: Direct weighing

iii. Use a clean scopula to transfer sample into container slowly, until you reach the desired mass.

Indirect Weighing

i. Place enough of the sample in a weighing bottle, put the lid on, and place on the scale. Record the mass.

ii. Take some out and place it in a different container (whatever you will be using for the experiment). Record the new mass. The difference in mass is the mass of the sample transferred.

iii. Continue this procedure until you have as much sample as you need.

iv. It is best to transfer small amounts at a time, so you do not take more than you need. You should not put excess sample back into the weighing bottle.

2. **Analytical balance:** Use the same procedure as with a toploader, remembering these additional points (Fig. 4.2)

i. Close all the doors before taking measurements.

ii. Remember the number of significant figures. It is higher than on a regular toploader.

iii. Make sure the sample is completely cooled when weighing. If a sample is still warm, it will weigh less because of buoyancy due to upward circulation of hot air.

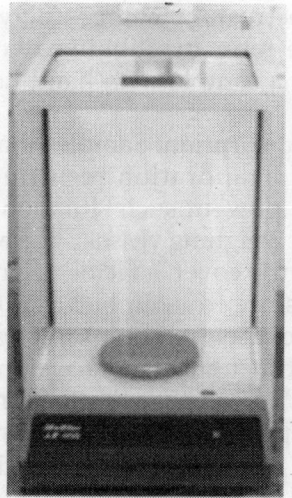

Fig. 4.2: An analytical balance

For example, a 50 ml beaker 3 minutes after removal from a 110° oven weighs 27.0271 g. At room temperature, it weighs 27.0410 g.

Possible Errors in Weighing

Oscillations: They are transmitted by the ground and walls, and the source that generates them are the devices and objects moving in communication course and the staff hence, the most successful method of preventing them, is to remove them from weighing process.

Vibrations: Vibrations are transmitted to balance mechanical system, so the most successful method of preventing them, is to remove them from weighing process.

Breeze of air: Balance workstation should not be located close to doors or windows. Closeness to devices, such as air-conditioning, fans, as well as places like communication courses should be avoided.

Fluctuation in temperature: Weighing room temperature should be maintained at constant level. Before analysis start, while performing it and after its finishing, temperature should be stable.

Electrostatics: Electrostatic charges may develop due to positive or negative ions, by rubbing two non-conducive substances, touching a sample with hand hence these things should be avoided.

Evaporation and absorption: Samples that are liquids, can undergo process of evaporation resulting in continuous decrease. In order to prevent such situations, liquid samples should be weighed in weighing vessels, like bulbs with narrow necks or vessels with top cover, a factor reverse to evaporation is absorption of moisture from ambient air by a sample. It is very important in case of hygroscopic samples. For the purpose of proper weighing of such substances, weighing vessel should be clean and dry. The easiest way to eliminate moisture absorption factor is application of hermetic vessels.

Magnetism: The electromagnetic field of a balance is disturbed or weighed sample is influenced by magnet installed in a balance. A solution for this problem is removal of a weighed sample from electromagnetic field of a balance, or by using special racks or hooks made of aluminum.

Minimum Weighing Amount

It is generally agreed that pharmaceutical products should be prepared with a *low percentage of error*. The official compendia allow a tolerance of ± 5% for most formulas, although greater accuracy may be required for very potent drugs with greater toxicity potential. This same degree of accuracy is expected in all extemporaneously compounded products.

Most pharmaceutical products allow for a tolerance of only **5% error**, where

$$\% \text{ Error} = \frac{\text{Error of measurement}}{\text{Quantity desired}} \times 100\%$$

If we know the sensitivity of the balance (i.e. the potential error) we can calculate the percentage of possible error when any amount of the substance is weighed.

$$\% \text{ Error} = \frac{\text{Sensitivity}}{\text{Quantity desired}} \times 100\%$$

For example, the Class III prescription balance has a sensitivity of 6 mg. What % of error would result in weighing 50 mg of a drug on the balance?

$$\% \text{ Error} = \frac{6 \text{ mg}}{50 \text{ mg}} \times 100\% = 12\%$$

Similarly, we can calculate the smallest quantity that can be weighed, on a balance of known sensitivity, to maintain a desired level of accuracy. This weight is referred to as the **least weighable quantity (LWQ)**.

$$\text{LWQ} = \frac{\text{Sensitivity}}{\% \text{ Error tolerated}} \times 100\%$$

For example, what is the least weighable quantity that will result in an error of 5% or less on a Class III prescription balance?

$$\text{LWQ} = \frac{6 \text{ mg}}{5\%} \times 100\% = 120 \text{ mg}$$

When a prescription formula calls for the incorporation of a component weighing less than 120 mg, special methods must be employed to obtain that weight of the component. If a liquid dosage form (solution, suspension or emulsion) is being prepared, the *liquid aliquot method* is employed. When the component must be incorporated as a solid into powders, tablets, capsules, or pastes, the *trituration method* is used.

Geometric Dilution

This method is used when potent substances are to be mixed with a large amount of diluent. Potent drugs are those drugs whose dose is less and diluents are substances which have no therapeutic effect and they are added to increase the volume of formulation. Geometric Dilution is the process by which a homogenous mixture or even distribution of two or more substances is achieved. When using this method, the smallest quantity of active ingredient is mixed thoroughly with an equal volume of the diluent. More diluents is added in amounts equal to the volume of the mixture. This process is repeated until all of the diluent is incorporated in the mixture. This method, though time consuming, will create a homogenous mixture.

For example, if 100 mg of potent drug is required to be mixed with 900 mg of lactose, then according to geometric dilution, the following procedure should be followed:

100 mg of a potent drug + 100 mg of lactose = 200 mg of mixture

200 mg of the mixture + 200 mg of lactose = 400 mg of mixture

400 mg of the mixture + 400 mg of lactose = 800 mg of mixture

800 mg of the mixture + remaining portion of lactose = 1000 mg of mixture.

ISOLATED KEY POINTS

- Topical powders usually contain starch or talc in addition to an active ingredient, such as an antifungal, antibacterial, or antipruritic agent.
- It is important to reduce the particle size of topical powders to produce a product that will be soothing to irritated skin.
- Powders are the solid dosage forms are available mostly in unit dosage forms, (consisting of doses which are taken by numbers) such as, tablets, capsules, pills, cachets or powders.
- A pharmaceutical powder is a mixture of finely divided drug and/or chemicals in dry form. These are solid dosage form of medicament which are meant for internal and external use
- Powders are classified as:
    - i. Bulk powder for external use
    - ii. Bulk powders for internal use
    - iii. Simple and compound powders
    - iv. Effervescent granules
    - v. Cachets.
- Effervescent powders are dispensed as single-dose or multidose preparations and generally contain acid substances and carbonates or hydrogen carbonates which react rapidly in the presence of water to release carbon dioxide.
- An efflorescent substance is a chemical which has water associated with its molecules, and which, when exposed to air, loses this water through evaporation.
- **Hygroscopic substances:** These are those substances which when exposed to environment absorb the moisture from the environment. Examples CaO, $NaNO_3$,
- Deliquescence, the process by which a substance absorbs moisture from the atmosphere until it dissolves in the absorbed water and forms a solution.
- **Eutectic mixtures:** When two or more substances are mixed together they liquefy due to the formation of a new

compound which has a lower melting point than room temperature.

- Geometric dilution is the process by which a homogenous mixture or even distribution of two or more substances is achieved. When using this method, the smallest quantity of active ingredient is mixed thoroughly with an equal volume of the diluent. More diluents is added in amounts equal to the volume of the mixture. This process is repeated until all of the diluent is incorporated in the mixture.

PRACTICE QUESTIONS
LONG ANSWER TYPE QUESTIONS

1. Define the term powder? Give advantages and disadvantages of powders?

2. Discuss in brief about simple and compound powders?

3. Give classification of powders? Enumerate various types of powders with suitable example in brief?

4. Write short notes on:
   a. Dusting powder
   b. Effervescent powder
   c. Hygroscopic powders

5. What do you mean by eutectic mixtures? Explain with the help of a suitable example.

6. What is geometric dilution? Give significance of geometric dilution for the formulation of potent drugs.

OBJECTIVE TYPE QUESTIONS

Multiple Choice question, select the best answer to the following statements.

1. The following procedure is used to reduce the particle size of powders:
   a. Trituration
   b. Geometric dilution
   c. Tumbling
   d. None of the above

2. Preparing a homogenous mixture of powders can be accomplished by:
   a. Spatulation
   b. Geometric dilution
   c. Tumbling
   d. All of the above

3. Which of the following powders would not be used as a diluent in a topical powder formulation.
   a. Starch
   b. Salicylic acid
   c. Talc
   d. None of the above

4. If the amount of an ingredient needed for a compounded solid dosage form is less than the minimum weighable quantity of the balance, the technician should:
   a. Call the prescriber and ask to change to a different ingredient
   b. Double all the ingredients and save half for the next refill
   c. Prepare an aliquot using the required ingredient and a diluent
   d. None of the above

TRUE/FALSE

Mark the following statements True (T) or False (F)

5. Bulk powders can be administered internally to dose antacids, bulk laxatives, and antidiarrheals ....

6. Trituration is one way to achieve comminution of dry powders ....

7. With a mesh sieve, the larger the mesh number, the larger the particles that can pass through it ....

8. In geometric dilution, the powder with the largest quantity is placed in the mortar and the powders with smaller quantities are added slowly; mixing is repeated after each addition ....

9. Bulk powders for internal use are sometimes called dusting powders ....

Answers

1. a   2. d   3. c   4. c   5. T   6. T
7. F   8. F   9. F

Chapter 5

Monophasic Liquid Dosage Form

These are the pharmaceutical dosage forms that are designed to provide maximum therapeutic response in population with difficulty of swallowing of tablets or capsules or to produce rapid therapeutic response. Water is the major ingredient used in these dosage forms. Maintenance of both physical and chemical stability of formulation is the main challenge in designing a liquid dosage form. Based on the physical characteristics, the liquid dosage form is divided into two types: Solutions and dispersed systems (suspensions and emulsions).

Excipients Used in Liquid Dosage Form

Excipients play an important role in formulating a dosage form. These are the ingredients which along with active pharmaceutical ingredients make up the dosage forms. In most of the formulations these are present in a greater proportion with regards to active pharmaceutical ingredient, as it forms about the bulk of the formulation, it is necessary to select an excipient which satisfies the ideal properties for a particular excipient. Pharmaceutical excipients are substances other than the pharmacologically active drug which are include in the manufacturing process or are contained in a finished pharmaceutical product dosage form. Excipients act as protective agents, bulking agents and can also be used to improve bioavailability of drugs in some instances. Excipients as like other active pharmaceutical ingredients need to be stabilized and standardized. Excipient quality plays a vital role in assuring safety, quality and efficacy of dosage forms.

VEHICLE

Vehicles, in pharmaceutical formulations, are the liquid bases that carry drugs and other excipients in dissolved or dispersed state. Pharmaceutical vehicles can be classified as under:

Aqueous vehicles: Water, hydro-alcoholic, polyhydric alcohols and buffers. These may be thin liquids, thick syrupy liquids, mucilages or hydrocolloidal bases.

Oily vehicles: Vegetable oils, mineral oils, organic oily bases or emulsified bases.

Water

Water is the most widely used vehicle in the preparation of pharmaceutical solutions. It acts as a universal solvent in solubilizing many active ingredients.

Advantages

   i. Widely available, inexpensive

  ii. Palatable

 iii. Non-toxic and non-irritable both for oral use and external use

 iv. Acts a solvent for many drugs.

Different types of water

Potable water: It is the normal drinking water that is palatable and safe for drinking. But this water is not used in the preparation of pharmaceutical dosage forms as they may contain microorganisms and the presence of dissolved mineral salts may contaminate the product.

Purified water: It is the water prepared from the potable water by distillation, by the use of ion exchange resin method, or by reverse osmosis.

Hard water: Hard waters are those that contain the Ca^{++} and Mg^{++} cations and alkaline waters are those that contain bicarbonates as the major impurity. These can be purified by using the above methods. To purify the water form micro-organisms, ultraviolet energy, heat or filtration (millipore filtration) methods can be used.

Distilled water: Distilled water is the purified water prepared by distillation process.

Freshly boiled and cooled water: This water is used for preparations intended for oral and external solutions. In this the boiling removes the dissolved gases like oxygen and CO_2 from the water. Stored water of this type is not used as it may act as source for contamination with microorganisms.

Aromatic waters: These are the clear saturated solutions of volatile oils, or other aromatic or volatile substances. These are mainly used as vehicles in oral solutions as they are flavoured or perfumed vehicles. These are generally prepared from concentrated ethanolic solution, in dilution with 1 part of concentrated water with 39 parts of water.

Chloroform water is a type of aromatic waters which adds sweetness to the preparation and also acts as a preservative. Some aromatic waters show mild carminative action, e.g. aromatic waters of Dill. Aromatic waters of volatile oils show salting out effect when a very soluble salt is added to the solution.

Water for injection: It is pyrogen free distilled water which is then sterilized and used in the preparation of parenteral solutions.

Alcohol (Ethyl Alcohol)

It is used as a primary solvent for many organic compounds. Alcohol has been well-recognized as a solvent and excipient in the formulation of oral pharmaceutical products. Next to water, alcohol is the most useful solvent in pharmacy. It is invariably used as hydro-alcoholic mixture that dissolves both water soluble and alcohol soluble drugs and excipients. Diluted alcohol NF, prepared by mixing equal volumes of Alcohol USP and purified water USP is a useful solvent in various pharmaceutical processes and formulations.

Glycerol

Glycerol (or Glycerin) is a clear, colourless liquid, with thick, syrupy consistence, oily to the touch, odourless, very sweet and slightly warm to the taste. When exposed to the air, it slowly abstracts moisture. It is miscible with both water and alcohol. As a solvent, it is comparable with alcohol but because of its viscosity, solutes are slowly soluble in it unless it is rendered less viscous by heating. Glycerol is obtained by the decomposition of vegetable or animal fats or fixed oils and containing not less than 95% of absolute glycerin. It is soluble in all proportions, in water or alcohol; also soluble in a mixture of 3 parts of alcohol and 1 part of ether, but insoluble in ether, chloroform, carbon disulphide, benzin, benzol, and fixed or volatile oils. Glycerin is used as vehicle in various pharmaceutical products like elixir of phosphoric acid, solution of ferric ammonium acetate, mucilage of tragacanth. As glycerin is an excellent solvent for numerous substances, such as iodine, bromine, alkalies, tannic acid, many neutral salts, alkaloids, salicin, etc., it is a good vehicle for applying these substances to the skin and to sores. It does not evaporate nor turn rancid, and is powerfully hygroscopic. As glycerin is sweet, it is an excellent flavouring agent. It is demulcent, and is used as a vehicle for applying substances, such as tannic acid, to the throat. In oral liquid formulations, glycerin is used as co-solvent to increase solubility of drugs that show low solubility in water. It is also used to improve viscosity, taste and flavour. In external applications it is used as humectants.

Propylene Glycol USP

Pharmaceutical grade of propylene glycol is monopropylene glycol (PG or MPG) with a specified purity greater than 99.8%. Propyleneglycol has become widely used as a solvent, extractant and preservative in a variety of parenteral and non-parenteral pharmaceutical formulations.

BUFFERING AGENTS

These are the agents which are added to maintain different ranges of pH of the solution. They resist the change in pH of the solution, e.g. Sorenson's modified phosphate buffer, sodium acetate buffer.

ISOTONICITY MODIFIERS

These are the agents added to maintain the isotonicity of the solutions similar to that of various body cavities. These are mainly added for ophthalmic solutions, injectable solutions and solutions applied for mucous membrane, e.g. dextrose and 0.9% NaCl solution.

VISCOSITY MODIFIERS

In order to increase the residence time of the aqueous based solutions that are intended for skin, eye, and ears, some jelling agents, in low concentrations are added to increase the viscosity of the product. Syrups may also be added to increase the viscosity of the product. They also improve palatability and ease pourability of the product, e.g. hydroxypropyl methycellulose, hydrroxyethyl cellulose, methylcellulose, polyvinyl alcohol, and polyvinyl pyrrolidine.

PRESERVATIVES

Preservatives are substances added to various pharmaceutical dosage forms and cosmetic preparations to prevent or inhibit microbial growth. An ideal preservative would be effective at low concentrations against all possible microorganism, be non-toxic and compatible with other constituent of the preparation and be stable for the shelf-life of the preparation.

 i. Ethanol (>10% v/v)
 ii. Propylene glycol (15–30% v/v)
 iii. Glycerin (>20% v/v)
 iv. Benzoic acid and sorbic acid (0.1% – 0.5% w/v)
 v. Chloroform water B. P. (0.25% v/v)
 vi. Methyl, ethyl, propyl and butyl parabens (up to 0.2%). These are stable over a pH range of 4 to 8. Generally combination of parabens is used in the formulations in order to achieve a higher total concentration and to be active against a wider range of microorganisms.
 vii. Quarternary ammonium compounds: Benzalkonium chloride (0.002–0.02%). It shows optimal activity over the pH range of 4 to 10. This shows incompatibility with most of anionic compounds due to its cationic nature.

ANTIOXIDANTS

Antioxidants are currently used as efficient excipients that delay or inhibit the oxidation process of molecules. These are agents used to prevent the products like vitamins, essential oils and fats from oxidation. The oxidation reaction may be due to heat, light and heavy metals. To prevent from heat and light they should be stored at cool temperature and in light resistance container respectively. EDTA or citric acid is mostly used to prevent oxidation by heavy metals like Fe, Cu., Other antioxidants: Ascorbic acid, citric acid, propyl and octyl estes of gallic acid, tocopherols, sodium metabisulfite, and sodium sulfite.

SWEETENING AGENTS

These are the agents added to mask the bitter taste of the active ingredient.

  i. Sucrose is widely used sweetening agent.

    a. *Advantages*: Colourless, highly water soluble, stable over a wide pH range (4–8), increase the viscosity, masks both salty and bitter taste, has soothing effect on throat.

    b. *Disadvantages*: Prolonged usage of the product with sucrose cause dental caries and it is also not suitable for diabetic patients.

  ii. Polyhydric alcohols, such as sorbitol, mannitol and glycerol also act as sweeteners and can be used for diabetic preparations.

FLAVOURS AND PERFUMES

These are the agents added to mask the unpleasant taste or odour and make the preparation more acceptable to take. Enable the easy identification of the product. For example, natural products like fruit juices (raspberry), extracts (liquorice), spirits (orange and lemon), syrups (black current), tinctures (ginger), and aromatic water (anise and cinnamon).

Some flavours are associated with special preparations, e.g. peppermint is associated with antacid preparations. Artificial perfumes are cheaper, more readily available and more stable than natural products.

COLOURING AGENTS

These are the agents added to enhance the appearance of the preparation. They should be non-toxic, non-irritant and should not show any therapeutic activity. Both natural and artificial coloring agents are available.

Natural colouring agents: These include materials extracted from plants and animals. Due to their low solubility mineral pigments like iron oxide are not added to the preparation, e.g. carotenoids, chlorophylls, saffron, red beet root extract, caramel, and cochineal.

Synthetic colours: Azo compounds. These are widely used as they give wide range of bright and stable colours.

WETTING AGENTS AND SURFACTANTS

Wetting agents are routinely used in pharmaceutical formulations, especially in liquid dosage forms to create a homogeneous dispersion of solid particles in a liquid vehicle. This process can be challenging due to a layer of adsorbed air on the particle's surface. Hence, even particles with a high density may float on the surface of the liquid until the air phase is displaced completely. The use of a wetting agent allows removal of adsorbed air and easy penetration of the liquid vehicle into pores of the particle in a short period of time. For an aqueous vehicle, alcohol, glycerin, and PG are frequently used to facilitate the removal of adsorbed air from the surface of particles. Whereas for a non-aqueous liquid vehicle, mineral oil is commonly used as a wetting agent. Typically, hydrophobic API particles are not easily wetted even after the removal of adsorbed air. Hence, it is necessary to reduce the interfacial tension between the particles and the liquid vehicle by using a surface active agent. For example, sodium lauryl sulfate is one of the most commonly used surface-active agents. Such surfactants, when dissolved in water, lower the contact angle of water and aid in spreadability of water on the particles surface to displace the air layer at the surface and replace it with the liquid phase. Wetting agents have a hydrophilic-lipophilic balance (HLB) value between 7 and 9.

METHODS TO ENHANCE THE SOLUBILITY

Solubility is the property of a solute to dissolve in a solvent to form a homogeneous solution. Any drug to be absorbed must be present in the form of solution. Most of the drugs are weakly acidic or weakly basic with poor water solubility. The solubility is commonly expressed as a concentration, either by mass (g of solute per kg of solvent, g per dL (100 ml) of solvent), molarity, molality, mole fraction, or other similar descriptions of concentration. (Table 5.1) All drugs have been divided into four classes.

A. Class I— High soluble and high permeable

B. Class II—High soluble and low permeable

C. Class III—Low soluble and high permeable

D. Class IV—Low soluble and low permeable

Table 5.1: USP and BP solubility criteria

Descriptive term	Part of solvent required per part of solute
Very soluble	Less than 1
Freely soluble	1 to 10
Sparingly soluble	30 to 100
Slightly soluble	100 to 1000
Very slightly soluble	1000 to 10,000
Practically insoluble	10,000 and over

Surfactants

Conventional approach to solubilize a poorly soluble substance is to reduce the interfacial tension between the surface of solute and solvent for better wetting and salvation interaction. A wide variety of surfactants like tweens, spans, polyoxyethylene stearates are very successful as excipient and carrier for dissolution enhancement.

Co-solvency

The solubility of a poorly water soluble drug can be increased frequently by the addition of a water miscible solvent in which the drug has good solubility known as co-solvents. Co-solvents are mixtures of water and one or more water miscible solvents used to create a solution with enhanced solubility for poorly soluble compounds. Examples of solvents used in co-solvent mixtures are PEG 300, propylene glycol or ethanol. Co-solvent formulations of poorly soluble drugs can be administered orally and parenterally. Poorly soluble compounds which are lipophilic or highly crystalline that have a high solubility in the solvent mixture may be suited to a co-solvent approach. Co-solvents can increase the solubility of poorly soluble compounds several thousand times compared to the aqueous solubility of the drug alone. The use of co-solvents is a highly effective technique to enhance the solubility of poorly soluble drugs. The most frequently used low toxicity co-solvents for are propylene glycol, ethanol, glycerin, and polyethylene glycol.

pH Adjustment

Poorly water soluble drugs with parts of the molecule that can be protonated (base) or deprotonated (acid) may potentially be dissolved in water by applying a pH change. pH adjustment can in principle be used for both oral and parenteral administration. In the stomach the pH is around 1 to 2 and in the duodenum the pH is between 5 and 7.5, so upon oral administration the degree of solubility is also likely be influenced as the drug passes through the intestines. Ionizable compounds that are stable and soluble after pH adjustment are best suited. The compound types may be acids or bases or zwitter ionic. It can also be applied to crystalline as well as lipophilic poorly soluble compounds. pH adjustment is also frequently combined with co-solvents to further increase the solubility of the poorly soluble drug. In situations where the drug precipitates into poorly soluble particles that require dissolution and do not rapidly redissolve.

MONOPHASIC LIQUIDS

Monophasic dosage forms are those liquid preparations in which there is only one phase and is represented by a true solution. A true solution is a clear homogeneous mixture which is prepared by dissolving a solid, liquid or gas (solute) in a suitable solvent. The solvent, or mixture of solvents, is the phase in which the dispersion occurs, and the solute is the component which is dispersed as molecules or ions in the solvent (Fig. 5.1).

Advantages

 i. Easier to swallow for children, old age, unconscious people.
 ii. Fast absorption since there is no need of dissolution.
 iii. Faster action than solid dosage forms.
 iv. Safe to administer substances like potassium iodide and bromide which cause gastric pain if taken in dry form.
 v. Can be administered via a number of routes like oral, parenteral preparations, topical (for use on the skin), otic (ear), nasal and ophthalmic preparations.

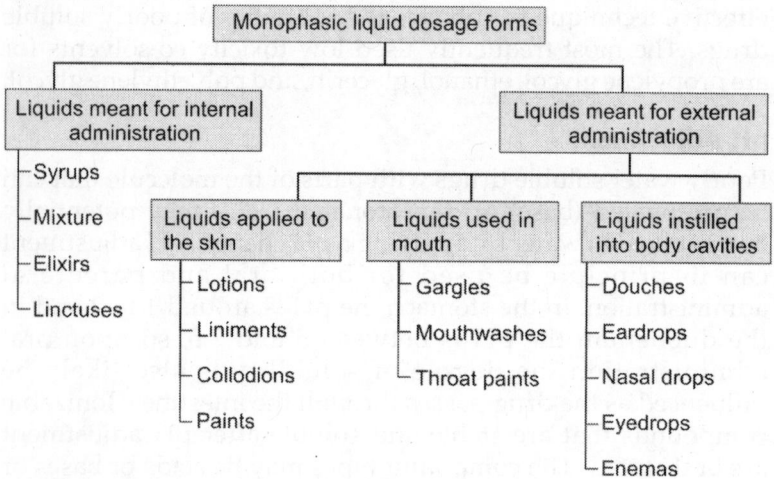

Fig. 5.1: Layout of classification of monophasic liquid dosage forms

Disadvantages

i. Bulky to carry

ii. Prone to microbial growth since contain water hence a preservative is required

iii. Solution can undergo hydrolysis when kept in direct sunlight, need special storage condition and must be labeled "Keep away from direct sunlight".

GARGLES

Gargles are aqueous and hydro alcoholic solution which is used to treat or prevent throat infection. They are dispensed in concentrated form with directions for dilution with warm water. They are brought into intimate contact with the mucous membrane of the throat and allow to remain for a few moments. They are used for deodourising and antibacterial effect.

They are usually available in concentrated form with direction for dilution with warm water before use. They are brought into intimate contact with the mucos membrane of the throat and are allowed to remain in contact with it for a few seconds, before they are thrown out of the mouth, they are used to relieve soreness in mild throat infection. It also stimulates secretion of saliva which relieves dryness, e.g. phenol gargles, potassium chloride and phenol gargles.

Storage: Store at room temperature keep out of the reach of children. Store away from direct sunlight, heat and moisture.

Labelling: The containers should be laelled "For external use only". The direction for proper dilution should be stated on the label.

Example: Prepare and dispense 100 ml of potassium chlorate and phenol gargle BPC.

Potassium chlorate and phenol gargles BPC.

Potassium chlorate	30.0 g
Patent blue V	0.009 g
Liquefied phenol	15.0 ml
Water sufficient to make	1000 ml

Method: Dissolve the potassium chlorate in warm water. Cool and add liqufied phenol. Add the dye solution, filter and make up volume. Transfer to a container, cork, label and dispense.

MOUTHWASHES

A mouthwash is an aqueous solution which is most often used for its deodorant, refreshing or antiseptic effect. It may contain alcohol, glycerin, synthetic sweeteners, surface-active agent, flavouring and colouring agents. Mouthwashes generally contain following substances:

1. Antibacterial agents: Alkaline phenol, hydrogen peroxide, buffered sodium perborate, thymol glycerin.
2. Astringents: Zinc sulphate, zinc chloride, etc.

Container: Narrow mouthed screw capped coloured fluted bottle.

Label: The label on the container should state—"Not to be swallowed in larges amount" and "Store in cool place and Dark place away from Sunlight".

Example: Prepare and dispense compound sodium chloride mouthwash.

R_x

Sodium bicarbonate	10 g
Sodium chloride	15 g
Concentrated peppermint emulsion	25 ml

Double strength chloroform water   500 ml
Purified water qs   1000 ml

Method of dispensing: Dissolve sodium bicarbonate and sodium chloride in purified water, add concentrated peppermint emulsion and mix. Add double strength chloroform water. Finally make up the volume with purified water.

Example: Prepare and dispense mouthwash.

R_x

Cetylpyridinium chloride	1 g
Citric acid	1 g
Sweetener (sodium saccharin)	0.4 g
Flavour oils (peppermint, eucalyptus and clove oils)	1.5 ml
Polyoxyethylene (20) sorbitan monostrate	3 g
Ethanol	100 ml
Sorbitol solution	200 g
Purified water (qs)	1000 ml

Method of dispensing: Dissolve cetylpyridinium chloride, citric acid and sodium saccharin in a sufficient amount of the water and add ethanol. Mix polyoxyethylene (20) sorbitan monostearate and flavour oils and add slowly hydroalcoholic solution with stirring, sorbitol and mix. Add sufficient amount of purified water to produce 1000 ml.

THROAT PAINTS

Throat paints are viscous liquid preparations used for mouth and throat infections. Glycerin is commonly used as a base because being viscous, it adheres to mucous membrane for a long period. It also provides a sweet taste to the preparation. The commonly used throat paints are boroglycerin, phenol glycerin, tannic acid glycerin, compound iodine paint (Mandl's paint).

Paints are solution or dispersions of one or more medicaments intended for application to the skin or, in some cases to the mucous membrane. They may contain volatile solvent that evaporates quickly to leave a dry or resinous film of medicament. Throat paints are more viscous due to high content of glycerin. Paints are sticky and adhere to the affected site and prolong the action of the medicament. Common example of paste are:

1. Brilliant green and crystal violet paints
2. Crystal violet paints

3. Coal tar paints
4. Mandl's paint
5. Tannic acid glycerin paints.

Storage: Paint should be kept in airtight containers.

Label: It should state "For external use only". Away from sunlight.

Container: "In a wide mouth screw capped bottles".

Example: Prepare and dispense brilliant green and crystal violet paint

R_x

Brilliant green	5 g
Crystal violet	5 g
Ethanol	500 ml
Purified water	1000 ml (qs)

Method of dispensing: Dissolve the brilliant green and crystal violet in ethanol (90%). Add sufficient water to produce 1000 ml.

Example: Prepare and dispense crystal violet paints.

R_x

Crystal violet	1 g
Purified water	1000 ml (qs)

Method of dispensing: Disperse the crystal violet in 700 ml of water and allow it to stand for one hour filter if necessary and make up the volume with water to 1000 ml.

Example: Prepare and dispense iodine paints (Mandl's paint)

In this preparation iodine act as antiseptic and potassium iodide dissolve the iodine, peppermint oil act as flavouring agent and produce cooling effect, alcohol is used as a solublizing agent for the peppermint oil. This preparation contains iodine, hence should be prepared id glass apparatus. It should not be prepared in mortar and pestle because porcelain contains pores and iodine enters in these pores. It is difficult to wash out the iodine and this entangled iodine can change the colour of other preparations.

R_x

Potassium iodide	25 g
Iodine	125 g
Ethanol (90%)	40 ml
Peppermint oil	4 ml
Purified water	25 ml
Glycerin	1000 ml (qs)

Method of dispensing: Dissolve potassium iodide and iodine in purified water in glass mortar and pestle with small portion of glycerin, add peppermint oil, dissolve in ethanol and mix. Add sufficient glycerin to produce 1000 ml.

EARDROPS

Ear preparations are liquid, semi-solid for instillation, for spraying or for insufflation, for application to the auditory meatus as an ear wash. Ear preparations usually contain one or more active substances in a suitable vehicle. They may contain excipients, e.g. to adjust tonicity or viscosity, to adjust or stabilize the pH, to increase the solubility of the active substances, to stabilize the preparation or to provide adequate antimicrobial properties. The excipients do not adversely affect the intended medicinal action of the preparation or, at the concentrations used, cause toxicity or undue local irritation.

Preparations for application to the injured ear, particularly where the eardrum is perforated, or prior to surgery is sterile, free from antimicrobial preservatives and supplied in single-dose containers. Ear preparations are supplied in multidose or single-dose containers, provided, if necessary, with a suitable administration device which may be designed to avoid the introduction of contaminants.

Example: Prepare and dispense 100 ml of soda glycerin.

R_x

Sodium bicarbonate	5 g
Glycerin	30 ml
Water (q.s)	100 ml

Method of preparation: Dissolve the sodium chloride in water add glycerin and mix it well. Finally make up the volume with water. Filter it, transfer it to a suitable container label it and dispense it. It is used to relieve itching in the ear and soften the wax.

Unless otherwise justified and authorized, aqueous ear preparations supplied in multidose containers contain a suitable antimicrobial or preservative. The ear preparations are of following types:

  i. Eardrops and sprays
 ii. Semi-solid ear preparations
iii. Ear powders
iv. Ear washes

In the manufacture, packaging, storage and distribution of ear preparations make sure to check for microbiological quality of pharmaceutical preparations. Sterile ear preparations are prepared using materials and methods designed to ensure sterility and to avoid the introduction of contaminants and the growth of microorganisms.

Storage: The preparation are stored in a sterile, airtight, tamper-proof container.

Labelling: The label should states:

i. The name of any added antimicrobial/preservative
ii. For multidose containers, the period after opening the container does not exceed 4 weeks, unless otherwise specified in pharmacopoeia.

NASAL DROPS

Drugs which are potent and required in lower doses, i.e. whose activity is required faster with fewer side effects, can be delivered through the nasal route. It is considered as one of the major route of drug administration to achieve faster and greater bioavailability of drug, as the nasal mucosa has high vasculature and high permeation of drugs.

Drugs are administered through nasal route for both topical effect and systemic effect. Topical administration includes delivery of drug to treat rhinitis, nasal congestion, sinusitis, and other related allergies. Most simple and convenient systems, but shows low dose precision. These are usually isotonic and slightly buffered to maintain a pH of 5.5 to 6.5. In addition appropriate antimicrobials and drug stabilizers are added if required, e.g. otrivine adult nasal drops 10 ml, Fenox nasal drops 15 ml, ephedrine nasal drops 0.5%.

Advantages

i. High permeability of nasal mucosa compared with epithelial tissue of GIT
ii. Rapid onset of action
iii. No first pass metabolism
iv. Potential for direct delivery to CNS
v. Avoidance of gastric irritation and vomiting
vi. Higher bioavailability of drugs than that of GIT.

Disadvantages

i. Sterility and stability problems

ii. Design of the device is difficult

iii. Difficult to use by pediatric and geriatric patients

iv. Dose is limited due to less available surface area.

Example: Prepare and dispense 100 ml of ephedrine nasal drops B.P.C

R_x

Ephedrine hydrochloride	0.5 g
Chlorobutol	0.5 g
Sodium chloride	0.5 g
Water (q.s)	1000 ml

Method of preparation: Dissolve the ephedrine hydrochloride, chlorbutol and sodium chloride in water, heat it. Cool it filter if necessary and make up the volume with water. Filter it, transfer it to a suitable container label it and dispense it.

ENEMA

Enemas are aqueous or oily solution or suspension or oil in water emulsion introduced into rectum or colon for cleansing (evacuation of feces) administration of nutrient substances, medicinal substances and opaque materials for radiological examination of lower intestinal tract.

Enemas are mostly used for the following reasons:

i. To relieve symptoms of constipation.

ii. To cleanse the rectum and lower intestines in preparation for an examination.

iii. To remove feces to prevent contamination during a surgical procedure.

iv. To administer anesthetic drugs to a patient.

Types of enemas: Enemas are of following types:

1. Cleansing enemas

2. Therapeutic enemas

3. Diagnostic enemas

4. Disposable enemas.

1. **Cleansing enemas:** Cleansing enemas used to evacuate feces in constipation or before an operation. They are of two types:
   i. By stimulating of peristalsis
      a. *Large volume*: Plain water, soft soap, turpentine enemas
      b. Small volume (osmotic retention) sodium phosphate enema, magnesium sulphate enema
      c. By lubricating impacted feces.

   Example are olive oil enemas, arachis oil enemas, glycerin enemas.

2. **Therapeutics enemas:** For sedative purpose like chloral hydrate paraldehyde and anti-inflammatory like corticosteroids.

3. **Diagnostic enemas:** It is used for X-ray examination of lower bowel. Example is barium sulphate enema.

4. **Disposable enemas:** Enemas available in disposable plastic bags.

They include evacuate enemas like magnesium sulphate retention enemas of prednisolone.

Containers: Single use plastic pack with rectal nozzle and label should state "To be warmed to body temperature before use".

SYRUPS

Syrups are concentrated oral solutions of sugar or nearly saturated solutions of sucrose in water or other aqueous liquids. Syrups containing 85% w/v or 66.7% w/w sucrose will retard the growth of microorganisms. Dilute solution of sucrose provides an excellent nutritional media for the growth of yeast, moulds and other microorganisms. When heat is employed for the preparation of syrups, a small portion of sucrose changes to dextrose and levulose. This phenomenon is called inversion. Sucrose solution is optically active and rotates polarized light to right while on heating optical activity decreases rotated the light to left due to formation of other compounds (dextrose ad levulose). The rate of inversion is enhanced by the presence of acids and hydrogen ions, which act as catalyst.

Syrups are mainly of three types:

1. **Simple syrup:** It contains sucrose in purified water alone or in combination of other polyols such as glycerin or sorbitol. These substances are added in syrups to reduce the crystallization of sucrose or improve the solubility of excipients.

2. **Medicated syrup:** It contains some added medicinal substances in the syrups and used for therapeutic purpose, e.g. ephedrine sulphate syrup.

3. **Flavoured syrup:** It contains various aromatic or pleasantly flavoured substances but are non-medicated and generally used as vehicle or as a flavouring agent or for preservation.

Methods of Preparation

Preparation of syrup depends on the physical and chemical characteristics of the substance employed for its preparation of syrups.

1. **Agitation without heat:** This method is used for the preparation of syrups containing volatile substances. In this process active medicament is added in solution and mixed in a glass-stopper bottle. For preparing large quantities, glass lined tank with mechanical agitators is employed. This method is used for the preparation of wide variety of syrups. Cough syrups are commonly prepared by this process, e.g. codeine syrup, ephedrine sulfate syrup, etc.

2. **Solution with heat:** This process is generally preferred as it is simple and less time consuming method, particularly if the constituents are not affected by heat and are non volatile in nature. In this process sucrose is added in the aqueous solution and heated till the sucrose is dissolved completely. Adding remaining amount of distilled water makes up volume of the solution. If the syrups containing any substances which are coagulated, it can be separated subsequently by straining. Excessive heating of syrup is not suitable because more inversion of sucrose occurs with the increase in temperature. Syrups cannot be sterilized in autoclave without caramelization. This solution is converted in yellowish to brown colour due to formation of caramel by the effect of heat on sucrose.

3. **Addition of a medicated liquid:** This method is used when other medicated substances in liquid form are added to syrup to medicate it. In this process some time precipitation takes place due to the presence of resinous and oily substances. It is necessary to take care that medicated substance should not get precipitated in this process.

4. **Percolation:** In this process, purified water or an aqueous solution is allowed to pass through a bed of crystalline sucrose. A plug of cotton is put in the neck of the percolator and purified water or aqueous solution is added in the percolator containing sucrose. The flow rate is controlled by the stopcock and maintained such that drops appear in rapid succession. If required, a small portion of liquid is re-passed through the percolator to dissolve the sugar completely in the liquid or aqueous solvent.

Preservatives

Syrup should be kept at low temperature, about 25°C is suitable for preservation. Preservatives are used to prevent bacterial and mould growth, viz. methyl paraben, propyl paraben, sodium benzoate, benzoic acid, etc.

Label and Storage

Syrup should be kept in well-closed containers and stored at temperature below 30°C. Bottle should be completely filled, carefully stoppered and stored in cool dark place.

Example: Prepare and dispense simple syrup

R_x

Sucrose	667 g
Purified water, sufficient to produce	1000 g

Or

R_x

Sucrose	850 g
Purified water, sufficient to produce	1000 ml

Example: Prepare and dispense invert syrup

R_x

Sucrose	66.7 g
Purified water, sufficient to produce	100.0 g

Hydrochloric acid   qs
Sodium carbonate as neutralizing agent

Method of Dispensing: Prepare syrup of sucrose 66.6% w/w in purified water and add hydrochloric acid slowly with continuous stirring. neutralize the solution using sodium carbonate solution

Example: Prepare and dispense Tolu syrup (1000 ml)

Rx

Tolu balsam	12.5 g
Sucrose	660 g
Purified water	1000 ml qs

Method of dispensing: Boil 400 ml of purified water in a vessel. Add weighed amount of tolu balsam in boiled water cover the vessel partially and boil the contents for 30 minutes. With frequently stirring add purified water to make contents of the vessel about to 360 g. Cool it and filter the solution add sucrose in the solution and warm it on a water bath to dissolve sucrose completely. Add sufficient water to make 1000 ml of the solution.

ELIXIRS

Elixirs are clear, flavoured hydroalcoholic preparation intended for oral use. They contain one or more medicament, pleasantly flavoured usually attractively coloured containing high proportion of alcohol or sucrose along with some suitable antimicrobial agent. The alcoholic content in elixir vary from 5–40%. In general they are more stable than mixture as sufficient alcohol is added to maintain the drug in the solution.

Elixirs are of two types:

1. **Non-medicated elixirs:** They are used purely as diluting agents or solvents for drugs containing approximately 25% alcohol, e.g. simple elixirs is alcoholic elixirs or low alcohol elixirs (containing 7–10% alcohol) high alcoholic elixirs (containing 60–75% alcohol).

2. **Medicated elixirs:** Elixirs containing therapeutically active compounds are known as medicated elixirs, e.g. phenobarbital elixirs US P, dexamethasone elixirs USP chlorpheniramine maleate elixirs.

The elixirs are generally marketed as ready to use like cough syrups, viz. dextromethorphan hydrobromide, codeine phosphate ammonium chloride. Some elixirs (phenethicillin and phenoxy methyl penicillin) are available in the market in granule or powder form because active ingredients are unstable in solution and there constituent will get degraded in presence of water. Hence, they are labelled as "Make up the volume up to the mark and shake well before use". The label also contain "store in a cool and dark place" and used the constituents within one week.

Example: Prepare and dispense high alcohol elixir

R_x

Compound orange spirit	4 ml
Saccharin	3 ml
Glycerin	200 ml
Alcohol	1000 ml (qs)

Method of dispensing: Dissolve the compound orange spirit and the Sacchrin in 70.0 ml of alcohol and glycerin. Add sufficient amount of alcohol to produce 100.0 ml and mix properly. Filter the mixture and preserve in suitable container.

Example: Prepare and dispense simple elixir

R_x

Orange tincture	75 ml
Syrup	400 ml
Chloroform water	1000 ml (qs)

Method of dispensing: Mix orange tincture with the syrup and add sufficient chloroform water to produce 100.0 ml. Add 5% of purified talc and shake vigorously. Filter the elixir and preserve in a sutaible container.

Example: Prepare and dispense pediatric paracetamol elixir

R_x

Paracetamol	24 ml
Ethanol (96%)	100 ml
Propylene glycol	100 ml
Concentrated raspberry juice	25 ml
Choloroformn spirit	20 ml
Inverrt syrup	275 ml
Amaranth solution	2 ml
Glycerin	1000 ml (qs)

Method of dispensing: Mix ethanol (96%), propylene glycol and choloroform spirit and make a mixture. Dissolve paracetamol and shake it, add other additives. Finally and sufficient amount of glycerin to produce 1000 ml.

Example: Prepare terpin hydrate elixir

R_x

Terpin hydrate	50 g
Orange oil	0.2 ml
Glycerin	400 ml
Alcohol	425 ml
Syrup	100 ml
Purified water	1000 ml (qs)

Method of dispensing: Dissolve terpin hydrate in alcohol and add other additives. Add sufficient purified water to produce 100 ml and mix if necessary, filter the elixir and preserve in a suitable container.

LINIMENTS

Liniments are solution or mixture of various substances in oil, alcoholic solution of soap or emulsions or occasionally semi-solid preparations intended for external application and should by labelled "For external use only". They are applied with rubbing or massaged into the skin as counter irritating or stimulating agents to the affected area.

Liniments are usually applied with friction and rubbing of the skin. The oil or soap base proving base of application and message. Alcoholic liniments are used generally for their rubifacient, counter irritant, mildly astringents and show penetrating effects. These types of liniments easily penetrate to the skin.

The oily liniments are slow in their action but are more useful when massaged. The function of liniment depends on the additives but most of liniments may function solely as protective coating on the affected area. Liniment should not be applied to the broken skin because they would be very irritating especially if alcohol is used as solvent.

They may contain following substances:

  a. Analgesic
  b. Antimicrobial
  c. Rubifacient
  d. Counter irritant

e. Stimulants
f. Soothing agents.

Although alcohol is primarily used as solvent, it enhances the penetration of the medicaments into the skin and has counter irritant or rubifacient action. Counter irritants are used to mask pain from fibrositis, sciatica, neuralgia and similar complaints by producing warmth, tingling and numbness. When rubbed onto the skin, they also cause redness and hence are called rubifacient. Cotton oil and arachis oil are less irritant than alcohol and spread more easily on the skin.

Two types of vehicle are used for the preparation of liniments (i) alchol, e.g. soap liniments and aconite liniments, and (ii) oils, e.g. camphor liniment and methyl salicylate liniment.

Labelling

It should be comply with the general requirements for labelling. In addition the labelling on the container should indicate—for external use only, shake well before use, not to be applied to wounds or broken skin, store in cool place.

Container

Narrow mouthed screw capped bottles can be used for dispensing liniments.

Example: Prepare and dispense white liniment

R_x

Oleic acid	85 ml
Turpentine oil	250 ml
Dilute ammonia solution	45 ml
Ammonium chloride	125 g
Purified water	1000 ml

Method of dispensing: Mix the oleic acid with measured quantity of turpentine oil. Mix dilute ammonia solution with 45 ml of purified water and warm it. Add warm diluted ammonia solution to the oily solution and shake to form an emulsion. Finally make up the volume with purified water.

Example: Prepare and dispense camphor liniment

R_x

Camphor	200 g
Arachis oil	800 g (qs)

Method of dispensing: Mix weighted amount of camphor in arachis oil in a closed vessel. Finally make up the volume with arachis oil

Example: Prepare and dispense soap liniment

R_x

Soft soap	10 g
Capmhor	10 g
Lemon grass oil	40 g
Purified water	15 ml
Alcohol (90.0%)	170 ml (qs)

Method of dispensing: Dissolve the weighted quantity of soap, camphor and lemon grass oil in alcohol. Add purified water and remaining amount of alcohol to make up the volume and mix.

Keep aside for a week and filter to remove the undissolved substance.

Example: Prepare and dispense turpentine liniment

R_x

Soft soap	50 g
Camphor	50 g
Turpentine oil	650 g
Purified water	1000 g (qs)

Method of dispensing: Mix the soft soap with small amount of purified water (100 ml). Make solution of camphor in fresh rectified turpentine oil. Gradually add camphor solution to the soap mixture with trituration until a thick creamy emulsion is formed. Finally add sufficient amount of purified water to make the volume and mix.

Example: Prepare and dispense calamine liniment

R_x

Calamine	50 g
Wool fat	10 g
Oleic acid	5 ml
Arachis oil	500 ml
Calcium hydroxide solution	1000 ml (qs)

Method of dispensing: Melt weighted amount of wool fat, oleic acid and arachis oil. Triturate calamine with melted oil. Add calcium hydroxide solution and shake it, transfer it to a suitable container and shake vigorously and finally make up the volume with calcium hydroxide solution.

LOTIONS

Lotions are usually liquid or liquid suspension or semi-solid preparations containing one or more medicaments, intended to be applied to the uniform skin without friction. They are lightly applied on the skin or applied on a suitable dressing and covered with waterproof substance like glycerin to reduce evaporation. They may be prepared by triturating the ingredients to a smooth paste and then gradually adding the remaining liquid phase. For large quantity preparation, high speed mixers or homogenizer are used. A wide variety of ingredients are employed in the preparation to produce better dispersions that show good cooling, soothing, drying or protective nature of the lotion. Following substances are used in the preparation of lotions.

1. **Bentonite:** As a suspending agent.
2. **Methylcellulose (MC) or sodium carboxymethylcellulose (Sodium CMC):** To hold the active ingredient in contact with the affected site.
3. **Glycerin:** Keep the skin moist for considerable period of time and to prevent the loss of moisture.
4. **Alcohol:** Used for increased the action like drying, cooling, etc.
5. **Miscellaneous:** Benzocaine, calamine, steroids, zinc oxide, etc.

Lotions are generally prescribed for the following purpose—anesthetic, antiseptic, astringent, germicide, protective, antihistaminic. Microorganisms may grow in certain lotions if no preservative is added. Care should be taken to avoid contamination during the preparation of lotion, even if it contains preservative.

Dilution of lotions: Care should be taken in dilution, particularly to prevent microbial contamination. The appropriate diluent should be used and heating should be avoided during mixing. Diluted lotions should be used within four weeks of their preparation.

Examples:

Acriflavine lotion	Dicholoroxylenol lotion	Salicylic acid lotion
Boric acid lotion	Gentian violet lotion	Thiomersal lotion
Calamine lotion	Oily calamine lotion	Zinc sulphate lotion
Cetrimide lotion	Dichloroxylenol lotion	Potassium permanganate lotion

Example: Prepare and dispense calamine lotion

R_x

Calamine	150 g
Zinc oxide	60 g
Bentonite	30 g
Sodium citrate	5 ml
Liquefied phenol	5 ml
Glycerin	50 ml
Rose water, sufficient to produce	1000 ml

Method of dispensing: Prepare sodium citrate solution in 700 ml rose water. Triturate calamine, zinc oxide, and bentonite with citrate solution in a mortar and pestle and add other additives and make sufficient volume with rose water.

Example: Prepare and dispense boric acid lotion

R_x

Chlorinated lime	12.5 g
Boric acid	12.5 g
Purified water, sufficient to produce	1000 ml

Method of dispensing: Mix chlorinated lime and boric acid and dissolve in purified water to produce 1000 ml.

Example: Prepare and dispense gentian violet lotion.

R_x

Gentian violet	10 g
Ethanol (95%)	100 ml
Purified water, sufficient to produce	1000 ml

Method of dispensing: Dissolve gentian violet in ethanol (95%) and add sufficient purified water to produce 1000 ml.

Containers: Narrow mouthed, fluted bottle.

Label: "Store in a cool and dry place away from sunlight" The label on the container should contain—'Shake well before use' and 'For external use only'.

ISOLATED KEY POINTS

- Monophasic dosage forms are those liquid preparations in which there is only one phase and is represented by a true solution.
- Gargles are aqueous and hydroalcoholic solution which is used to treat or prevent throat infection. They are dispensed

in concentrated form with directions for dilution with warm water.

- Mouthwash is an aqueous solution which is most often used for its deodorant, refreshing or antiseptic effect.
- Throat paints are viscous liquid preparations used for mouth and throat infections.
- Eardrops are liquid, semi-solid for instillation, for spraying or for insufflation, for application to the auditory meatus as an ear wash.
- Nasal drops are administered through nasal route for both topical effect and systemic effect.
- Enemas are aqueous or oily solution or suspension or oil in water emulsion introduced into rectum or colon for cleansing (evacuation of feces) administration of nutrient substances, medicinal substances and opaque materials for radiological examination of lower intestinal tract.
- Syrups are concentrated oral solutions of sugar or nearly saturated solutions of sucrose in water or other aqueous liquids containing 85% w/v or 66.7% w/w sucrose.
- Simple syrup contains sucrose in purified water alone or in combination of other polyols, such as glycerin or sorbitol. These substances are added in syrups to reduce the crystallization of sucrose or improve the solubility of excipients.
- Medicated syrup contains some added medicinal substances in the syrups and used for therapeutic purpose, e.g. ephedrine sulphate syrup.
- Flavoured syrup contains various aromatic or pleasantly flavoured substances but are non-medicated and generally used as vehicle or as a flavouring agent or for preservation.
- Elixirs are clear, flavoured hydroalcoholic preparation intended for oral use. They contain one or more medicament, pleasantly flavoured usually attractively coloured containing high proportion of alcohol or sucrose along with some suitable antimicrobial agent.
- Non-medicated elixirs contains approximately 25% alcohol, e.g. simple elixirs is alcoholic elixirs or low alcohol elixirs (containing 7–10% alcohol) high alcoholic elixirs (containing 60–75% alcohol).

- Medicated elixirs contains therapeutically active compounds are known as medicated elixirs, e.g. phenobarbital elixirs USP.
- Liniments are solution or mixture of various substances in oil, alcoholic solution of soap or emulsions or occasionally semisolid preparations intended for external application and should by labelled "For external use only".
- Lotions are usually liquid or liquid suspension or semisolid preparations containing one or more medicaments, intended to be applied to the uniform skin without friction.

PRACTICE QUESTIONS
LONG ANSWER TYPE QUESTION

1. What are monophasic liquid dosage form? Give advantages and disadvantages of monophasic liquid dosage form.
2. Compare and contrast between gargle and mouthwash.
3. Write short notes on:
   a. Gargle
   b. Mouthwash
   c. Throat paint
4. What are syrups? Give there method of preparation in detail.
5. Write in details about elixir with the help of suitable examples.
6. Write short notes on:
   a. Liniments
   b. Lotions
7. Define the term otic products. What are the various factors which is to be kept in mind in designing the otic dosage form?
8. What are nasal products? Give their advantages and disadvantages.

OBJECTIVE TYPE QUESTIONS

1. Nasal formulations are generally administered in volumes ranging from ....

2. Which of the following is not true for nasal drug delivery system:
   a. Drugs are administered for both topical effect and systemic effect
   b. Drugs administer include corticosteroids, anticholinergics, antihistamines, etc.
   c. Drug administer give fastest and highest bioavailability
   d. Used to administer drugs that are ineffective orally, small dose requirement and need rapid systemic absorption

3. Which of the following is advantage in respect to nasal drug delivery system:
   a. No first pass metabolism
   b. No sterility and stability problems
   c. Design of the device is easy
   d. Easy to use by pediatric and geriatric patients

4. The pH of a nasal formulation is important for the following reasons:
   a. To avoid irritation of nasal mucosa
   b. To allow the drug to be available in unionized form for absorption
   c. To prevent growth of pathogenic bacteria in the nasal passage
   d. To sustain normal physiological ciliary movement

Answers

1. 25 to 200 μL　　　2. c　　　3. a　　　4. a

Chapter 6

Biphasic Liquids Emulsion and Suspension

EMULSION

A **Pharmaceutical emulsion** is a two-phase liquid preparation consisting of two or more immiscible liquids in which small globules of one liquid are dispersed uniformly throughout the other liquid. The liquid that is dispersed as small globules is called the dispersed phase or external phase or discontinuous phase and the other liquid is called the dispersion medium or external phase or continuous phase.

Emulsion is a thermodynamically unstable liquid preparation containing at least two immiscible liquids, in which one liquid phase is dispersed as globules (dispersed or internal phase) in other liquid phase (continuous or external phase) stabilized with the aid of an emulsifying agent (Fig. 6.1). General types of pharmaceutical emulsions include lotions, liniments, ointments, creams, and vitamin drops.

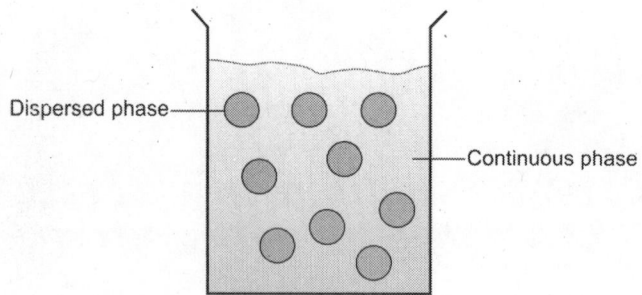

Dispersed phase

Continuous phase

Fig. 6.1: Dispersed phase and continuous phase of an emulsion

Advantages and Disadvantages of Emulsions

Advantages

i. Unpalatable drugs can be administered in palatable form.

ii. Oil sensation of oil soluble drugs can be masked as aqueous phase can easily disperses the flavours in it.

iii. Improve the rate of absorption of drugs.

iv. Two incompatible ingredients can be included one in each phase of an emulsion.

Disadvantages

i. The emulsion should be shaked every time prior to administration

ii. It needs an accurate measuring device for measuring the dose for administration

iii. Proper storage conditions are required

iv. Bulky and difficult to transport and may prone to breakage

v. Easily contaminated by microorganisms that leads to emulsion instability.

TYPES OF EMULSIONS

1. Macroemulsion or simple emulsion
2. Microemulsion
3. Multiple emulsion

1. Macroemulsions (simple emulsions): In this type of emulsion one phase of emulsion gets dispersed in the other phase generally water in oil (w/o type) or oil in water (o/w type) (Table 6.1 and Fig. 6.2). The size of the droplets is approximately 5 µm.

Oil in water (o/w): In this the oil droplets are dispersed in a continuous aqueous phase. This emulsion is generally formed if the aqueous phase constitutes more than 45% of the total weight. In this a hydrophilic emulsifier is used. The globule size is 0.25 to 10 microns. These are generally used for oral administration. These are useful as water washable drug bases.

Water in oil (w/o): In this the aqueous phase is dispersed in a continuous oily phase. This emulsion is generally formed if the oily phase constitutes more than 45% of the total weight and a lipophobic emulsifier is used. These are generally used

Pharmaceutics II

for cosmetics. These are employed for treatment of dry skin and emollient applications (Table 6.1).

Table 6.1: Difference between o/w and w/o Emulsions

S. No	Oil in water emulsion (o/w)	Water in oil emulsion (w/o)
1.	Water is the dispersion medium and oil is the dispersed phase	Oil is the dispersion medium and water is the dispersed phase
2.	They are non greasy and easily removable from the skin surface	They are greasy and not water washable
3.	They are used externally to provide cooling effect, e.g. vanishing cream	They are used externally to prevent evaporation of moisture from the surface of skin, e.g. cold cream
4.	Water soluble drugs are more quickly released from o/w emulsions	Oil soluble drugs are more quickly released from w/o emulsions
5.	They are preferred for formulations meant for internal use as bitter taste of oils can be masked	They are preferred for formulations meant for external use like creams
6.	O/w emulsions give a positive conductivity test as water is the external phase which is a good conductor of electricity	W/o emulsions go not give a positive conductivity test as oil is the external phase which is a poor conductor of electricity

Emulsion o/w (oil/water)   Emulsion w/o (water/oil)

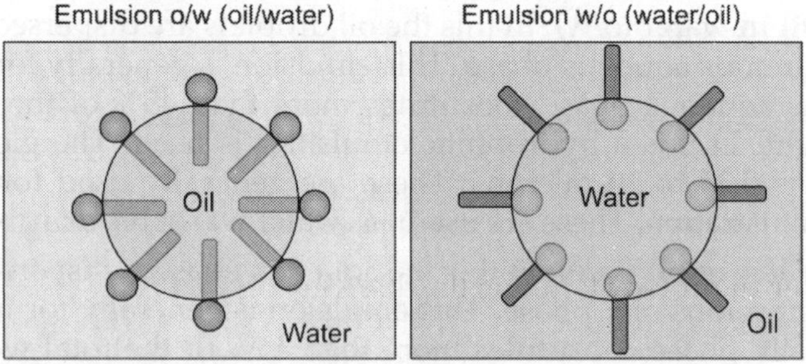

Fig. 6.2: A simple emulsion: O/w type and w/o type

2. Microemulsions: These are the clear, homogenous emulsions in which one insoluble liquid is dispersed in a second liquid. Droplets size range 0.01 to 0.1 µm. These are generally referred to as solubilized systems or transparent emulsions, micellar solutions as they appear as true solutions to the naked eye. Microemulsions are believed to be thermodynamically stable. These are used for drug administration and toiletry products.

Pharmaceutical Applications of Microemulsions

 i. Increases the bioavailability of poorly water soluble drugs.
 ii. Topical drug delivery systems.

3. Multiple emulsions: These emulsions consist of three phases that are developed with a view to delay the release of an active ingredient. They may be oil-in-water-in-oil (o/w/o) or of water-in-oil-in-water (w/o/w) (Fig. 6.3). Lipophilic (oil-soluble, low HLB) surfactants are used to stabilize w/o emulsions, whereas hydrophilic (water-soluble, high HLB) surfactants are used to stabilize o/w systems. In these type of emulsions the drug is present in innermost phase so that is has to cross two phase boundaries to reach the external continuous phase. In some cases inversion of such emulsions take place such that they form simple emulsions by converting from a w/o/w emulsion to o/w emulsion.

Preparation of Multiple Emulsions

In this the aqueous phase is added to oily phase, containing a lipophilic surfactant by continuous mixing. This results in the

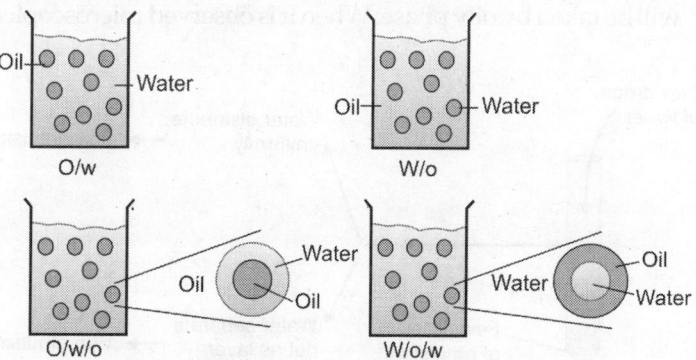

Fig. 6.3: Multiple emulsions

formation of primary w/o emulsion. This w/o emulsion is then poured into a second aqueous solution that has a hydrophilic surfactant by continuous mixing. This results in the formation of a w/o/w multiple emulsion.

Pharmaceutical applications:

i. Multiple emulsions are widely used in cosmetics, pharmaceuticals and foods.

ii. They sustained the release of active ingredient as it has to pass from the internal phase (w/o or o/w phase) to the continuous phase (either water or oil). They can also improve dissolutions or solubilization of insoluble materials.

iii. These types of emulsions are used to protect sensitive and active molecules, such as vitamin C and E from undergoing antioxidation.

TEST FOR IDENTIFICATION OF EMULSION

1. Dilution test: In general the emulsion will be diluted only with its continuous phase. Hence o/w can be diluted with water and w/o can be diluted with oil. So when oil is added to o/w emulsion or when water is added to w/o emulsion, separation of internal and continuous phase occurs. This test is used for liquid emulsions (Fig. 6.4).

2. Dye solubility test: In general water soluble dye (e.g. amaranth dye or methylene blue) will be taken up by the aqueous phase whereas oil soluble dye (e.g. Scarlet dye) will be taken by oily phase. When it is observed microscopically

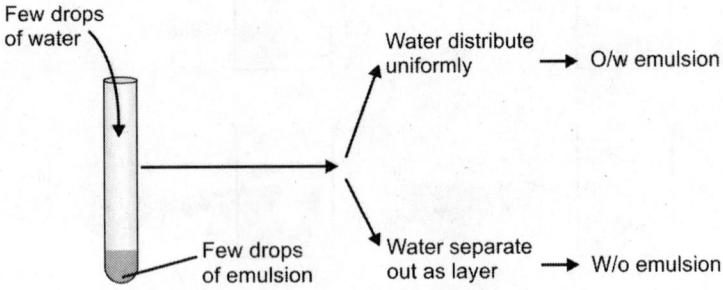

Fig 6.4: Dilution test for liquid emulsions

that water soluble dye is taken up by the continuous phase, it is o/w emulsion. If the dye is not taken up by the continuous phase, test is repeated with oil soluble dye. If it is taken up by the continuous phase, it can be confirmed as w/o emulsion. This test can fail if ionic emulsions are present (Fig. 6.5).

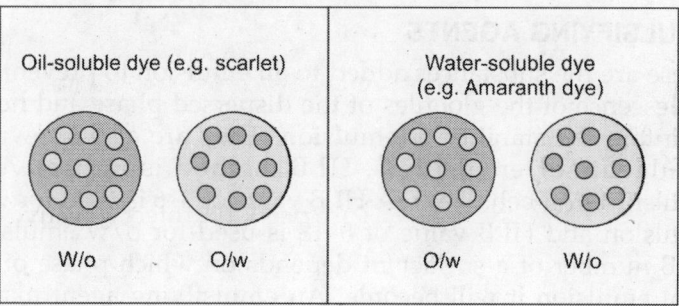

Fig. 6.5: Microscopic examination of type of emulsion by dye solubility test

3. **Conductivity test:** Water is a good conductor of electricity whereas oil is non conductor of electricity. When a pair of electrodes connected to a lamp and an electrical source are dipped into emulsion and on pressing the key the bulb glows it means the given emulsion is o/w type emulsion and if the lamp does not light, it means the given emulsion is w/o type emulsion (Fig. 6.6).

4. **CoCl$_2$ filter test:** To a filter paper impregnated with CoCl$_2$ and dried (blue), o/w emulsion is added. It changes to pink.

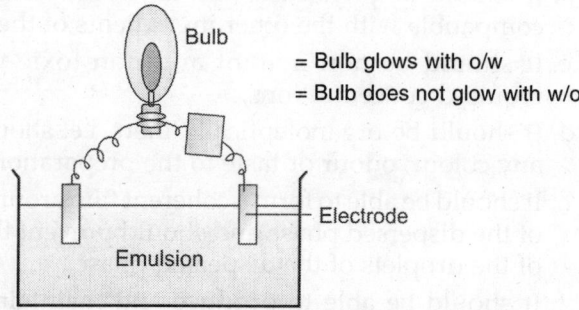

Fig. 6.6: Conductivity test for determination of type of emulsion

It may fail if emulsion is unstable or breaks in presence of electrolyte.

5. **Fluorescence test:** Since some oils fluoresce under UV light, o/w emulsions exhibit no fluorescence whereas w/o emulsion exhibits fluoresce. But this test is applicable for oils that have fluorescent property.

EMULSIFYING AGENTS

These are the substances added to an emulsion to prevent the coalescence of the globules of the dispersed phase and hence maintain the stability of emulsion. They are also known as emulgents or emulsifiers. HLB method is indicative of emulsification behaviour. A HLB value of 3–6 is used for w/o emulsion and HLB value of 8–18 is used for o/w emulsion. HLB number of a surfactant depends on which phase of the final emulsion it will become. An emulsifying agent mainly acts by the following mechanisms:

i. **Reduction in interfacial tension:** Thermodynamic stabilization

ii. **Formation of a rigid interfacial film:** Mechanical barrier to coalescence

iii. **Formation of an electrical double layer:** Repulsion of individual droplets.

Ideal Requirements of Emulsifying Agent

a. It should be able to reduce the interfacial tension between the two immiscible liquids.

b. It should be physically and chemically stable, inert and compatible with the other ingredients of the formulation.

c. It should be non irritant and non toxic when used in required concentrations.

d. It should be organoleptically inert, i.e. should not impart any colour, odour or taste to the preparation.

e. It should be able to form a coherent film around the globules of the dispersed phase and should prevent the coalescence of the droplets of the dispersed phase.

f. It should be able to produce and maintain the required viscosity of the preparation.

Classification of Emulsifying Agents

a. Synthetic surface active agents (monomolecular films)

b. Semi synthetic polysaccharides

c. Natural hydrophilic colloids (multimolecular films)

d. Finely divided solid particles (particulate film)

e. Auxiliary emulsifying agents.

Synthetic Surface Active Agents

This group contains surface active agents which act by getting adsorbed at the oil water interface in such a way that the hydrophilic polar groups are oriented towards water and lipophilic non polar groups are oriented towards oil, thus forming a stable film. This film acts as a mechanical barrier and thus prevents coalescence of the globules of the dispersed phase. The functions of surface active agents to provide stability to dispersed droplets are as following:

i. Reduction of the interfacial tension

ii. Form coherent monolayer to prevent the coalescence of two droplet when they approach each other (Fig. 6.7)

iii. Provide surface charge which cause repulsion between adjacent particles.

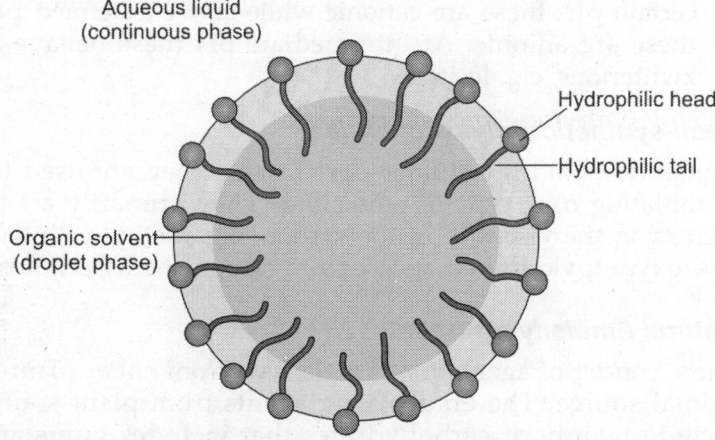

Fig. 6.7: Formation of monomolecular film by surface active agent

Classification of synthetic surface active agents: They are classified according to the ionic charge possessed by the molecules of the surfactant.

I. **Anionic surfactants:** These agents are primarily used for external preparations and not for internal use as they have an unpleasant bitter taste and irritant action on the intestinal mucosa, e.g. alkali soaps, polyvalent soaps (metallic soaps), organic soaps, sulfated alcohols and alkyl sulfonates.

II. **Cationic surfactants:** They are mainly used in external preparations, such as lotions and creams. They have good antibacterial activity and are also used in combination with secondary emulsifying agents to produce o/w emulsions for external application, e.g. quaternary ammonium compounds, such as cetrimide, benzalkonium chloride and benzethonium chloride.

III. **Non-ionic surfactants:** These are widely used as emulsifying agents to prepare both w/o and o/w emulsions for internal as well as external use, e.g. glyceryl esters, polyoxyethylene glycol esters and ethers, sorbitan fatty acid esters (spans), polyoxyethylene derivatives of sorbitan fatty acid esters (tweens or polysorbates), polyoxyethylene/polyoxypropylene block polymers (poloxamers).

IV. **Ampholytic surfactants:** These are the substances whose ionic charge depends on the pH of the system. Below a certain pH, these are cationic while above a defined pH, these are anionic. At intermediate pH these behave as zwitterions, e.g. lecithin.

Semi-synthetic Polysaccharides

It mainly includes cellulose derivatives. They are used for formulating o/w type of emulsions. They primarily act by increasing the viscosity of the system, e.g. methyl cellulose, hydroxypropylcellulose and sodium carboxymethylcellulose.

Natural Emulsifying Agents

These consist of agents that are derived from either plant or animal source. The emulsifying agents from plant source include mainly of carbohydrates that includes gums and mucilaginous substances. They act as primary emulsifying agents as well as secondary emulsifying agents (emulsion stabilizers). Since carbohydrates acts a good medium for the growth of microorganism, the emulsions prepared using these emulsifying agents have to be suitably preserved in order to prevent microbial contamination, e.g. tragacanth, acacia, agar, chondrus (Irish Moss), pectin and starch. The emulsifying agents from animal source include lecithin, cholesterol and wool fat.

Finely Dispersed Solids

They form particulate films around the dispersed droplets and produce coarse grained emulsions that are stable, e.g. colloidal clays like bentonite, veegum (magnesium aluminium silicate, magnesium trisilicate, metallic hydroxides, magnesium hydroxide and aluminium hydroxide.

Auxiliary (Secondary) Emulsifying Agents

Auxiliary emulsifying agents include those compounds that are normally incapable themselves to form stable emulsion. Their main value lies in their ability to function as thickening agents and thereby helping to stabilize the emulsion. They increase the viscosity of the external phase and restrict the collision of droplets. Some of them prevent coalescence by reducing van der waals forces between particles or by providing a physical barrier between droplets. Proteins, semisynthetic polysaccharides (methylcellulose, carboxymethylcellulose), clays can be used as auxiliary agents.

METHOD OF PREPARATION OF EMULSION

While preparing the acacia emulsions for extemporaneous use, primary emulsion formula must be used. Based on the nature of the oil different formulas are there (Table 6.2).

Preparation techniques of emulsions: The preparation techniques for emulsion can be divided into laboratory scale productions and large-scale productions.

Laboratory scale techniques: Techniques used on laboratory scale are:
1. Continental or dry gum method
2. Wet gum method

Table 6.2: Formula for preparation of primary emulsion

Nature of oil	Examples	Oil	Water	Gum
		Ratios of ingredients		
Fixed oil	Castor oil, almond oil, arachis oil	4	2	1
Mineral oil	Liquid paraffin	3	2	1
Volatile oil	Turpentine oil, peppermint oil	2	2	1
Oleo gum resin	Male fern extract	1	2	1

3. Bottle or forbes bottle method
4. Auxiliary method
5. *In situ* soap method.

Continental method or dry gum method: The continental method is used to prepare the initial or primary emulsion from oil, water and an emulsifier (gum usually acacia) in 4:2:1 ratio. The 4 parts of oil and 1 part of gum represent their total amount for the final emulsion.

Method: In this 1 part of gum (acacia) is triturated with 4 parts of oil in a motor, until the powder is thoroughly wetted. Then 2 parts of water is added all at once and the mixture is vigorously and continuously triturated until a creamy white primary emulsion is formed. Additional water may be incorporated after the primary emulsion is formed. Solid substances (like active ingredients, preservatives, colors and flavours) are added as a solution to the primary emulsion, oil soluble substances in small amounts may be incorporated directly into the primary emulsion. Any substance which might reduce the physical stability of the emulsion, such as alcohol (which may precipitate the gum) is added at the end of the in order to avoid breaking the emulsion. When all agents have been incorporated, the emulsion should be transferred to a calibrated vessel, and the final volume is made with water, then homogenized or blended to ensure uniform distribution of ingredients.

Example: Cod liver oil emulsion

Cod liver oil	50 ml
Acacia	12.5 g
Syrup	10 ml

| Flavour oil | 0.4 ml |
| Purified oil | up to 100 ml |

Method: Weigh accurately all the ingredients. The cod liver oil is placed in dry mortar. Add acacia and mix it quickly. Add 25 ml of water and immediately triturate to form thick white, homogenous primary emulsion. Add flavour and mix. Add syrup and mix. Add sufficient water to make the final volume.

Wet gum method or English method: In this method the proportion of oil and water and emulsifier (gum) are in the ratio of 4:2:1, but the order and technique of mixing is different from dry gum method. In this 1 part of gum is triturated with 2 parts of water to form mucilage. To these four parts of oil is slowly added in portions, while triturating. After all the oil is added, the mixture is triturated for several minutes to form the primary emulsion. Then other ingredients are added as in continental method. In general the English method is more difficult to perform successfully, especially with more viscous oils, but it results in a more stable emulsion.

Bottle method: This method is used to prepare emulsions with volatile oils, or oleaginous substances of very low viscosities. This method is a variation of dry gum method. One part of powdered acacia (or other gum) is placed in a dry bottle and 4 parts of oil are added. The bottle is capped and thoroughly shaken. The time of mixing the gum and oil should be less as the gum will tend to imbibe the oil and will become waterproof. To this required volume of water is added all at once and shaked thoroughly until the primary emulsion is formed.

Auxiliary method: A hand homogenizer is used to improve the emulsion prepared by other methods. In this the emulsion is passed through a very small orifice, and hence reduces the dispersed droplet size to about 5 microns or less.

In situ **soap method:** This contains oils, such as olive oil, oleic acid along with lime water (calcium hydroxide solution, USP). These are called calcium soaps. It is prepared by mixing equal volumes of oil and lime water.

Example: Nascent soap which consists of oil phase as olive oil/oleic acid and lime water as aqueous phase. Olive oil can be replaced by other oils but oleic acid must be added. Lime water [$Ca(OH)_2$] should be freshly prepared. The emulsion formed is w/o type emulsion.

STABILITY PROBLEMS OF EMULSION

Physical instability: The physical instability of the emulsion can be assessed by the following phenomenon (Fig. 6.8):

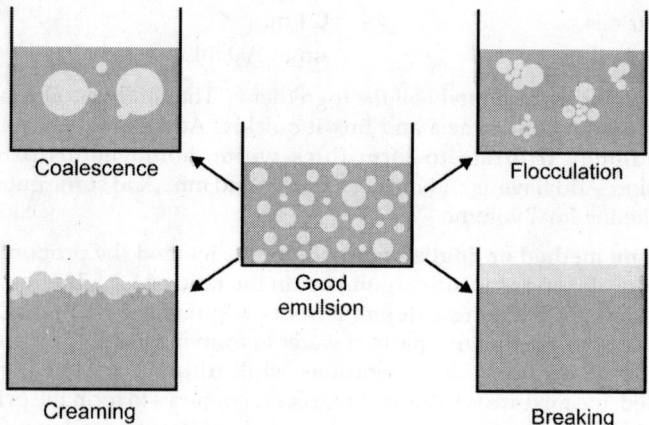

Fig. 6.8: Physical instability of an emulsion

1. Cracking
2. Flocculation
3. Creaming and sedimentation
4. Breaking
5. Phase inversion

1. Coalescence (cracking): In this, the emulsified globules join to form larger particles. The major factor which prevents coalescence is the mechanical strength of electrical barrier. This can be prevented by the addition of natural gums as auxiliary emulsifiers at low concentrations.

Reasons for coalescence (cracking)

Globule size: If globule size is more 1–3 μm, creaming of emulsion takes place followed by cracking. Hence globule size is reduced.

Storage temperature: Extremes of temperature leads to cracking. Freezing of water causes undue pressure on dispersed globules and the emulsifying film that leads to cracking. On the other hand, increase in temperature decreases the viscosity of the continuous phase and disrupts the integrity of interfacial film. An increasing number of collisions between droplets will also occur, leading to increased creaming and cracking.

2. Flocculation: Flocculation is defined as the association of globules within an emulsion to form large aggregates. However, these aggregates can easily be redispersed upon shaking. It is considered as a precursor to the irreversible coalescence. It differs from coalescence mainly in that interfacial film and individual droplets remain intact. Flocculation is influenced by the charges on the surface of the emulsified globules. The reversibility of flocculation depends upon strength of interaction between particles as determined by:

i. The chemical nature of emulsifier
ii. The phase volume ratio
iii. The concentration of dissolved substances, specially electrolytes and ionic emulsifiers.

3. Creaming and sedimentation: The upward or downward movement of dispersed droplets is termed creaming and sedimentation respectively. In any emulsion, creaming or sedimentation takes place depending on the densities of dispersed and continuous phases. Creaming or sedimentation is undesirable as it may lead to coalescence.

Rate of creaming of emulsion: The rate of creaming of an emulsion is governed by Stoke's law. It is given by the following equation:

$$Y = 2r^2 (\rho_1 - \rho_2) \, g/9\eta$$

where,

Y = Rate of creaming or sedimentation
r = Radius of droplets of dispersed phase
ρ_1, ρ_2 = Density of dispersed and continuous phase respectively
g = Gravitational rate constant
η = Viscosity of continuous phase.

Factors affecting rate of creaming

Droplet size: As per Stoke's law, rate of creaming is directly proportional to the square of radius of the globule or droplet. Smaller is the diameter of the droplet, lesser will be the rate of creaming. Hence reduction in droplet size helps in reducing creaming or sedimentation.

Difference in densities of dispersed and continuous phase: As per Stoke's law creaming is avoided if densities of the two phases are equal and it can be achieved by adjusting the density of dispersed phase.

Viscosity of the continuous phase: As per Stoke's law, rate of creaming is inversely proportional to viscosity of the continuous phase. Hence increase in viscosity of the continuous phase by viscosity enhancing agents reduces the rate of creaming.

Viscosity of continuous phase: Clays and gums increase the viscosity of continuous phase. For w/o emulsions addition of polyvalent metal soaps or high melting waxes and resins in the oil phase can be used to increase the viscosity.

Volume of internal phase: More the volume of internal phase greater is the viscosity.

Particle size of dispersed phase: Smaller the globule size more will be the viscosity and hence enhanced stability of emulsion can be achieved by reduction in globule size.

4. Breaking: It occurs due to coalescence and creaming of an emulsion which results in the complete separation of the oil from the water so that it floats at the top in a single, continuous layer.

5. Phase inversion: Conversion of one type of emulsion to other type (like w/o type to o/w type and vice versa) is termed phase inversion. The optimum range of concentration of the dispersed phase should be 30–60% of the total volume. If this range exceeds to about 74%, it may result in inversion of the emulsion. Other factors leading to phase inversion are:

    a. Temperature of the system: Increased temperature of o/w (with polyoxyethylenated nonionic surfactant) makes the emulsifier more hydrophobic and the emulsion may invert to w/o type.

    b. Addition of strong electrolytes to o/w emulsion (stabilized by ionic surfactants) may invert to w/o emulsion, e.g. addition of polyvalent Ca ions leads to inversion of o/w emulsion (stabilized by sodium cetyl sulfate and cholesterol) to a w/o type emulsion.

PARAMETERS FOR ASSESSING THE EMULSION STABILITY

Both physical and chemical parameters are used to assess emulsion stability.

Physical parameters: The following parameters are commonly measured to assess the effect of stress conditions on emulsions.

1. Phase separation
2. Viscosity
3. Electrophoretic properties
   i. Zeta potential
   ii. Electrical conductivity
   iii. Dielectric constant
4. Particle size distribution analysis

1. Phase separation: The rate and extent of phase separation after aging of an emulsion may be observed visually or by measuring the volume of separated phase. The separated phase may be due to coalescence or due to creaming. It is important to differentiate between the coalescence and creaming, since the means of correcting these defects are different. To detect this small samples of the emulsion are withdrawn from top and the bottom of the preparation after some period of storage and the composition of the two samples are compared by appropriate analysis of water content, oil content or any other suitable constituent.

2. Viscosity: Changes in viscosity during aging can give an idea about shelf-life of an emulsion. Viscometers of cone and plate type or instruments having co-axial cylinders are used to measure the viscosity. The viscosity changes in first few days are different for w/o and o/w emulsions. The viscosity of w/o emulsion decreases up to certain period (5–15 days) and then remains constant. This is due to the formation of floccules by the oil globules. In case of o/w emulsions flocculation causes increase in viscosity for some time. After this initial change almost all emulsions show changes in consistency with time, which follow a linear relationship on a log scale. The complete absence of slope (no change in viscosity with age) is ideal. However, slight increase of viscosity between 0.04 and 400 days is acceptable. Other emulsions exhibit much more drastic and sudden nonlinear increases in viscosity after two to three months aging. Such behaviour is frequently followed by a drop in viscosity probably associated with phase inversion.

Pharmaceutics II

3. **Electrophoretic properties:** The following electrophoretic properties are to be determined to evaluate emulsion stability.

   a. *Zeta potential:* Stability of emulsions can be evaluated through zeta potential measurement by evaluating the effect of the repulsive forces between globules. It is observed that a minimum zeta potential of ± 50 mV is needed to get satisfactory stability of dispersion. Zeta potential of emulsion is useful for assessing flocculation since electrical charges on particles influence the rate of flocculation. Reduction of zeta potential on aging indicates instability of the emulsion. Maximum zeta potential is associated with maximum emulsion stability.

   b. *Electrical conductivity:* It is also used to evaluate emulsion stability. The electrical conductivity of o/w or w/o emulsions is determined using platinum electrodes for a short-time at room temperature or at 37°C. Conductivity depends on degree of dispersion. O/w emulsions with fine particles exhibit low resistance. If resistance increases, it is a sign of aggregation and instability. A fine emulsion of water in w/o product does not conduct current until droplet coagulation occurs which indicates instability of emulsion.

   c. *Dielectric constant:* An inverse relationship existed between log of rate of increase in dielectric constant and the absolute temperature. This can be used as a prediction test.

4. **Particle size distribution analysis:** Particle size is inversely proportional to the stability. Changes of the average particle size or size distribution of droplets are important parameters for evaluating emulsion stability. Particle analysis can be carried out by microscopic methods or by electronic counting devices, e.g. coulter counter method.

PACKAGING OF EMULSIONS

These are generally packaged in wide mouthed containers made of plastic, glass and metal. Parenteral emulsions are generally stored in glass vials or glass ampoules or glass bottles. Disposable syringes are generally made of plastic material. The stoppers used are made up of elastomeric materials. Metallic containers are used for packaging of topical emulsions. This protects the emulsion from light. The following Table 6.3 represents the type of packaging of pharmaceutical emulsions.

Table 6.3: Packaging of pharmaceutical emulsions

Emulsion type	Bottle type	Typical size
Oral emulsions	Amber flat medical bottles	50 ml, 100 ml, 150 ml, 200 ml, 300 ml and 500 ml
External emulsions	Amber fluted medical bottles	50 ml, 100 ml and 200 ml

Expiry date of emulsions: The expiry date of oral emulsion is for 4 weeks if no guidance is available. The preparation should be discarded after the expiry date.

Labelling requirements of emulsions: The labelling of pharmaceutical emulsions is important for ease of patient administration. They are as follows.

i. Shake well before use

ii. For external use only: In case of external emulsions that are not intended for oral use.

iii. Do not freeze

iv. Protect from direct sunlight.

SUSPENSIONS

Suspensions are class of liquid dosage forms in which the finely divided solid particles (internal phase) are dispersed uniformly in a liquid dispersion medium (external phase). The internal phase consisting of insoluble solid particles having a range of size (0.5 to 5 microns) which is maintained uniformly throughout the suspending vehicle with aid of single or combination of suspending agent. The external phase (suspending medium) is generally aqueous in some cases it may be an organic or oily liquid for non oral use. The formulation, manufacturing, stability and packaging are the important aspects to be considered in the designing of pharmaceutical suspensions.

Advantages and Disadvantages of Suspension

Advantages

i. Insoluble derivatives of certain drugs are more palatable than soluble forms and these derivatives are formulated in the form of suspensions.

ii. Some insoluble derivatives of drugs are more stable in aqueous solvents than in the soluble salts.

iii. Suspension can improve chemical stability of certain drug. For example, procaine penicillin G.

iv. Suspended insoluble powders are easy to swallow. Bulky powders such as kaolin BP and chalk BP can be administered in suspension form which acts as adsorbents of toxic substances in the gastrointestinal tract.

v. Drug in suspension exhibits higher rate of bioavailability than other solid dosage forms. The decreasing order of bioavailability of drug in the dosage form is as follows:

   a. Solution > Suspension > Capsule > Compressed Tablet > Coated tablet

vi. Duration and onset of action can be control, e.g. protamine zinc-insulin suspension.

vii. Suspension can mask the unpleasant/bitter taste of dreg, e.g. chloramphenicol palmitate.

Disadvantages

i. They should be shaked well prior to administration.

ii. Physical stability, sedimentation and compaction can causes problems.

iii. Care should be taken while handling and transport due to its bulky nature.

iv. Formulation of an ideal suspension is difficult.

v. Uniform and accurate dose cannot be achieved unless suspension is packed in single dosage form.

Desired Features of an Ideal Pharmaceutical Suspension

a. The sediment formed should be easily re-suspended by the use of moderate shaking.

b. It should be easy to pour.

c. It should have pleasant odour, colour and palatability.

d. It should have good syringeability.

e. It should be physically, chemically and microbiologically stable.

f. Parenteral/ophthalmic suspension should be sterile.

CLASSIFICATION OF SUSPENSIONS

Based on Route of Administration

a. Oral suspensions

b. Parenteral suspensions

c. Topical suspensions.

Based on Proportion of Solid Particles

a. Dilute suspension (2 to 10% w/v solid)

b. Concentrated suspension (50% w/v solid).

Based on Electrokinetic Nature of Solid Particles

a. Flocculated suspension

b. Deflocculated suspension.

Based on Size of Solid Particles

a. Colloidal suspension (< 1 micron)

b. Coarse suspension (>1 micron).

Reasons for the formulation of a pharmaceutical suspension:

i. The drug is insoluble in the vehicle.

ii. To mask the bitter taste of the drug

iii. To increase the stability of the drug

iv. To make the drug sustained or controlled release.

Method of Preparation

The preparation of suspension includes three methods:

1. Use of controlled flocculation

2. Use of structured vehicle

3. Combination of both, i.e. use of controlled flocculation and structured vehicle.

IMPORTANT CONSIDERATIONS IN FORMULATION OF A SUSPENSION

During the formulation of a suspension, the properties both the dispersed phase and dispersion medium should be known well in order to obtain a good suspension (Flowchart 6.1). The route of administration, intended application and possible adverse effects of the material should be well-studied, and then it is selected for formulating into a suspension. The following are the most important factors that are to be considered during formulation a pharmaceutical suspension.

Nature of the suspended material: The suspended particles should possess low interfacial tension so that they are easily wetted by water and hence can be suspended easily. Particles with high interfacial tension are not wetted easily. In this case surfactants are used which reduces the interfacial tension of the particles and increases their wettability.

Size of the suspended particles: As per the Stroke's law, the sedimentation rate decreases when the particle size is reduced. It is given by the equation:

$$\text{Rate of sedimentation, } V = \frac{d2(\rho_1 - \rho_2)g}{18\eta_0}$$

Flowchart: 6.1: Method of preparation of suspension

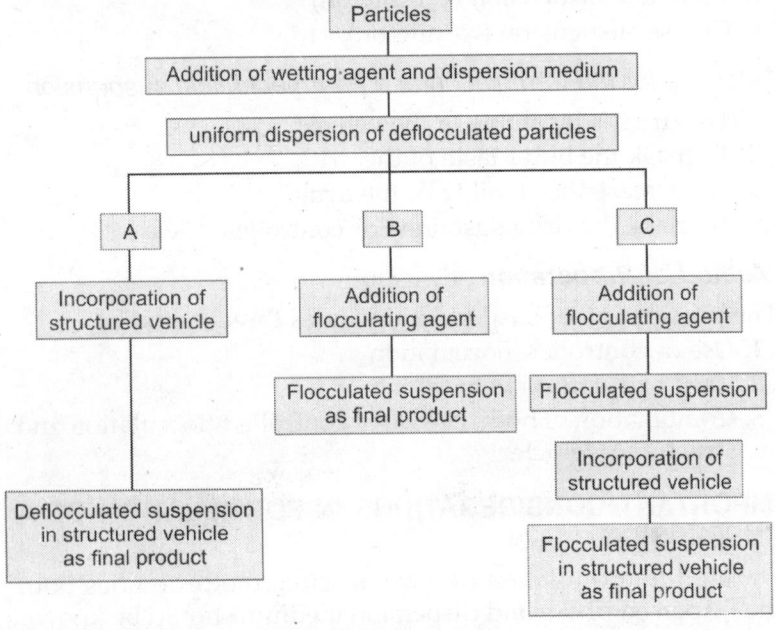

where,

V = Terminal velocity of sedimentation (cm/s)

d = Diameter of the particle (cm)

η_0 = Viscosity of the suspending medium

g = Acceleration due to gravity

ρ_1 and ρ_2 = Densities of the suspending particles and the medium respectively.

Factors Affecting Sedimentation

Particle size diameter (d): Sedimentation velocity (v) is directly proportional to the square of diameter of particle (d).

$$V \propto d^2$$

Density difference between dispersed phase and dispersion media ($\rho_1 - \rho_2$): The velocity of sedimentation is directly proportional to the difference between the dispersed phase and dispersion medium.

$$V \propto (\rho_1 - \rho_2)$$

Generally, the density of the suspended particles is greater than dispersion medium. But in certain cases particle density is less than dispersion medium, so suspended particle floats and hence uniform dispersion of the particles is difficult. If density of the dispersed phase and dispersion medium are equal, the rate of settling becomes zero.

Viscosity of dispersion medium (η_0): Sedimentation velocity is inversely proportional to viscosity of dispersion medium.

$$V \propto 1/\eta_0$$

Increase in viscosity of medium decreases settling, so that the particles achieve good dispersion system. But increase in viscosity should be not be such that it gives rise to problems like pouring, syringeability and redispersibility of suspension.

Sedimentation parameters: There are two important parameters that are to be considered in the formulation of suspensions.

i. Sedimentation volume (F)

ii. Degree of flocculation (B)

Sedimentation volume (F): It is the ratio of final or ultimate volume (V_u) of the sediment to original volume of the suspension (V_O). The sedimentation volume gives only a qualitative account of suspension. It is given by the equation;

$$F = V_u/V_O$$

Sometimes sedimentation volume is represented as height of suspension (H) when measuring cylinder is used to measure the volume of sediment. It is given by the equation;

$$F = Hu/Ho$$

where,

    Hu = Final or ultimate height of the sediment;

    Ho = Initial or original height of the sediment;

The following diagrammatic representation (Fig. 6.9) shows the sedimentation volumes of flocculated and deflocculated suspensions.

Ranges of Sedimentation Volume

    i. Sedimentation volume can have values ranging from < 1 to > 1

    ii. F is normally less than 1.

    iii. When $F = 1$, the suspension is said to be in flocculation equilibrium and it shows no clear supernatant on standing. It is said as an Ideal Suspension.

Degree of flocculation (β): It is the ratio of ultimate volume of sedimentation (F) of the flocculated suspension to the ultimate volume of sedimentation (F_∞) of the deflocculated suspension.

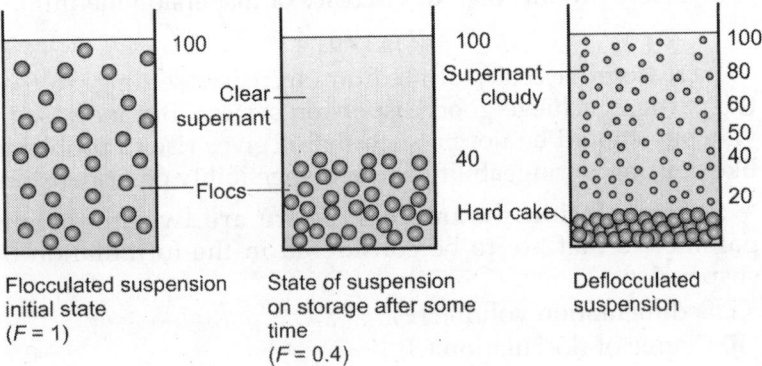

Flocculated suspension initial state $(F = 1)$ State of suspension on storage after some time $(F = 0.4)$ Deflocculated suspension

Fig. 6.9: Sedimentation volume of flocculated and deflocculated suspensions

Degree of flocculation, $\beta = F/F_\infty$

Applications of Pharmaceutical Suspensions

1. Suspension is usually applicable for drug which is insoluble or poorly soluble, e.g. prednisolone.
2. To enhance the stability of drug, e.g. oxytetracycline suspension.
3. To mask bitter or unpleasant taste of the drug, e.g. chloramphenicol palmitate suspension.
4. Suspension of drug can be formulated for topical application, e.g. calamine lotion.
5. Suspension can be formulated for parenteral application in order to control rate of drug absorption, e.g. procaine penicillin.
6. Vaccines are often formulated as suspension, e.g. cholera vaccine.
7. X-ray contrast agents can also be formulated as suspension, e.g. barium sulfate for examination of alimentary tract.

FLOCCULATED AND DEFLOCCULATED SUSPENSION

Flocculated Suspensions

In flocculated suspension, formed flocs (loose aggregates) will cause increase in sedimentation rate due to increase in size of sedimenting particles. Hence, flocculated suspensions sediment more rapidly. Here, the sedimentation depends not only on the size of the flocs but also on the porosity of flocs.

Deflocculated Suspensions

In deflocculated suspension, individual particles are settling. Rate of sedimentation is slow, which prevents entrapping of liquid medium which makes it difficult to re-disperse by agitation. This phenomenon called 'caking' or 'claying'. In deflocculated suspension larger particles settle fast and smaller remain in supernatant liquid so supernatant appears cloudy (Table 6.4).

The Sedimentation Behaviour of Flocculated and Deflocculated Suspensions

Flocculated suspensions: In the flocculated suspension, the flocks or loose aggregates formed increases the rate of

Table 6.4: Difference between flocculated and deflocculated suspension

Flocculated	Deflocculated
1. Particles forms loose aggregates and form a network like structure	1. Particles exist as separate entities
2. Rate of sedimentation is high	2. Rate of sedimentation is slow
3. Sediment is rapidly formed	3. Sediment is slowly formed
4. Sediment is loosely packed and does not form a hard cake	4. Sediment is very closely packed and a hard cake is formed
5. Sediment is easy to redisperse	5. Sediment is difficult to redisperse
6. Suspension is not pleasing in appearance	6. Suspension is pleasing in appearance
7. The floccules stick to the sides of the bottle	7. They do not stick to the sides of the bottle

sedimentation of particles. Hence, the sediment will form at a faster rate. In this the sedimentation depends not only on the size of the flocks but also on the porosity of flocks. In this the loose structure of the rapidly sedimenting flocks tends to preserve in the sediment, which contains an appreciable amount of entrapped liquid (Fig. 6.10). In this case the volume of the final sediment is relatively large. This type of suspensions is easily redispersed upon little agitation.

Deflocculated suspensions: In deflocculated suspension, the particles of the suspension settle separately without formation of any flocks or aggregates. In the rate of sedimentation is slow that prevents entrapping of liquid medium in between the particles and hence, it forms a hard cake upon standing for longer period. The sediment cannot be redispersed by little agitation. This phenomenon is also called 'cracking' or 'claying'. In deflocculated suspension larger particles settles faster and the smaller particles remain in supernatant liquid. Hence supernatant appears cloudy. Whereas in flocculated suspension as the smaller particles are also involved in formation of flocks or aggregates, the supernatant does not appear cloudy.

STABILITY PROBLEMS WITH SUSPENSION

The following are some problems which are associated with the stability of suspension during their storage and shelf-life.

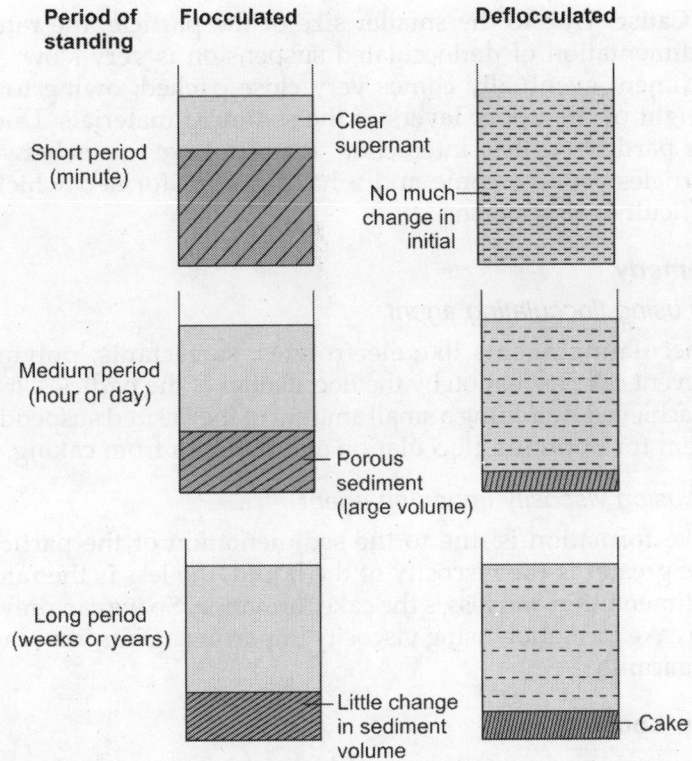

Fig. 6.10: Rate of sedimentation of flocculated and deflocculated suspension

1. Caking and poor redispersibility
2. Cap locking
3. Colour change
4. Crystal growth
5. Deflocculation
6. Rapid settling
7. Change in particle size
8. Foaming.

Caking and Poor Redispersibility

Caking is a compact mass of insoluble solids particle formed generally in deflocculated suspension.

Cause: Due to the smaller size of the particle, the rate of sedimentation of deflocculated suspension is very slow. The sediment eventually comes very close packed, owing to the weight of the upper layers of the sediment materials. Due to the particle-particle interaction, the repulsive forces between particles are overcome and a hard cake is formed which is difficult to redisperse.

Remedy

By using flocculating agent

Flocculating agents like electrolytes, surfactants, polymers prevent cake formation by the flocculation of the particles. It can be achieved by adding a small amount of the desired suspending agent for optimum flocculation and freedom from caking.

By using viscosity imparting agent

Cake formation is due to the sedimentation of the particles. The greater is the viscosity of the liquid, the less is the rate of sedimentation and less is the cake formation. So we can prevent the cake formation using viscosity imparting agents like acacia, tragacanth.

Cap Locking

Cap locking is a filling problem which occurs when the dispersed particles crystallize on the threads of the bottle cap and interface in cap removal.

Remedy: Cap locking can be prevented by using different vehicle containing sucrose, glucose.

Colour Change

Light sensitive colour may be changed in presence of light, due to the increased in surface area some color may be changed.

Remedy: Storing in cool and dark place.

Crystal Growth

Sometimes there is crystal growth during storage which can be due to following reasons.
   i. Fluctuation in temperature
   ii. Change in pH

iii. Due to impurities
iv. Poor solubility.

Remedy

  i. By adding surfactants
 ii. By controlling solubility
iii. By controlling pH
iv. By preventing temperature fluctuation.

Deflocculation

Deflocculation takes place due to following reasons:
  i. Change in pH
 ii. Adding of excess electrolytes
iii. Due to drug degradation.

Remedy

  i. By using flocculating agent
 ii. By using electrolytes
iii. By using polymer.

Rapid Settling

Some suspension particles settle fast.

Remedy

  i. By decreasing the particle size
 ii. By using viscosity imparting agents.

Change in Particle Size

Sometimes the particle size may be changed. Generally particle size is increased. Increased particle size leads to rapid settling.

Remedy

By using viscosity imparting agents.

Foaming

If the density of the particle is less than the density of the liquid medium, the negative velocity of the particle results, this is the rate of floating or creaming.

Remedy

By changing the aqueous phase.

ISOLATED KEY POINTS

- An emulsion is mixture of two liquids that would not normally mix. That is to say, a mixture of two immiscible liquids. By definition, an emulsion contains tiny particles of one liquid suspended in another.
- Emulsion types oil-in-water (o/w) water-in-oil (w/o) oil-in-water-in-oil (o/w/o) water-in-oil-in-water (w/o/w) determination of o/w or w/o water soluble dye (e.g. methylene blue) dilution of emulsions conduction of current.
- Physical stability of emulsion creaming is the upward movement of dispersed droplets of emulsion relative to the continuous phase (due to the density difference between two phases.
- Physical stability of emulsion breaking, coalescence, aggregation. Breaking is the destroying of the film surrounding the particles. Coalescence is the process by which emulsified particles merge with each to form large particles. Aggregation: dispersed particles come together but do not fuse. The major fact preventing coalescence is the mechanical strength of the interfacial film.
- Physical stability of emulsion phase inversion an emulsion is said to invert when it changes from an o/w to w/o or vice versa. Addition of electrolyte Addition of $CaCl_2$ into o/w emulsion formed by sodium stearate can be inverted to w/o. Changing the phase: volume ratio.
- **Methods of emulsion preparation:** Dry gum method the continental method is used to prepare the initial or primary emulsion from oil, water, and a hydrocolloid or "gum" type emulsifier (usually acacia). The primary emulsion, or emulsion nucleus, is formed from 4 parts oil, 2 parts water, and 1 part emulsifier.
- **Wet gum method:** In this method, the proportions of oil, water, and emulsifier are the same (4:2:1), but the order and techniques of mixing are different. The 1 part gum is triturated with 2 parts water to form a mucilage; then the 4 parts oil is added slowly, in portions, while triturating.

- **Bottle method:** This method may be used to prepare emulsions of volatile oils, or oleaginous substances of very low viscosities.

- Auxiliary method an emulsion prepared by other methods can also usually be improved by passing it through a hand homogenizer, which forces the emulsion through a very small orifice, reducing the dispersed droplet size to about 5 microns or less.

- **Microemulsion:** Microemulsions are thermodynamically stable, optically transparent, isotropic mixtures of a biophasic oil-water system stabilized with surfactants.

- **Pharmaceutical suspension:** A Pharmaceutical suspension is a coarse dispersion in which internal phase is dispersed uniformly throughout the external phase. The internal phase consisting of insoluble solid particles having a specific range of size which is maintained uniformly throughout the suspending vehicle with aid of single or combination of suspending agent. The external phase (suspending medium) is generally aqueous in some instance, may be an organic or oily liquid for non oral use.

- Classification; 1. based on general classes oral suspension—externally applied suspension, parenteral suspension; 2. Based on proportion of solid particles—dilute suspension (2 to 10% w/v solid), concentrated suspension (50% w/v solid); 3. Based on electrokinetic nature of solid particles—flocculated suspension, deflocculated suspension; 4. Based on size of solid particles—colloidal suspension (< 1 micron), coarse suspension (>1 micron) and nano suspension (10 ng).

- Advantages suspension can improve chemical stability of certain drug. Bioavailability is in following order, solution > suspension > capsule > compressed tablet > coated tablet duration and onset of action can be controlled, e.g. protamine zinc-insulin suspension can mask the unpleasant/bitter taste of drug, e.g. chloramphenicol palmitate.

- Disadvantages physical stability, sedimentation and compaction can causes problems. It is bulky sufficient care must be taken during handling and transport. It is difficult to formulate uniform and accurate dose cannot be achieved unless suspension are packed in unit dosage form.

- Theory of suspensions by stoke's equation $V = 2r^2 (\rho s - \rho o) g/9\eta$ where, V sed. = Sedimentation velocity in cm/sec d = Diameter of particle r = Radius of particle ρs = Density of disperse phase ρo = Density of disperse media g = Acceleration due to gravity η = Viscosity of disperse medium.

- Factors affecting sedimentation particle size radius (r) $V \propto r^2$. Density difference between dispersed phase and dispersion media $(\rho s - \rho o)$ $V \propto (\rho s - \rho o)$ generally, particle density is greater than dispersion medium but, in certain cases particle density is less than dispersed phase, so suspended particle floats and is difficult to distribute uniformly in the vehicle. If density of the dispersed phase and dispersion medium are equal, the rate of settling becomes zero.

- **The sedimentation behaviour of flocculated and deflocculated suspensions:** In flocculated suspension, formed flocks (loose aggregates) will cause increase in sedimentation rate due to increase in size of sedimenting particles. Hence, flocculated suspensions sediment more rapidly. Here, the sedimentation depends not only on the size of the flocs but also on the porosity of flocks. In flocculated suspension the loose structure of the rapidly sedimenting flocs tends to preserve in the sediment, which contains an appreciable amount of entrapped liquid. The volume of final sediment is thus relatively large and is easily redispersed by agitation.

- Deflocculated suspensions in deflocculated suspension, individual particles are settling, so rate of sedimentation is slow which prevents entrapping of liquid medium which makes it difficult to re-disperse by agitation.

- Flocculating agents decreases zeta potential of the suspended charged particle and thus cause aggregation (flock formation) of the particles. Examples of flocculating agents are: Neutral electrolytes, such as KCl, NaCl. Surfactants polymeric flocculating agents sulfate, citrates, phosphates salts.

- Viscosity of suspensions is of great importance for stability and pourability of suspensions.

- Different approaches to increase the viscosity of suspensions. Few of them are as follows, viscosity enhancers some natural gums (acacia, tragacanth), cellulose derivatives (sodium CMC, methyl cellulose), clays (bentonite, veegum), carbomers, colloidal silicon dioxide (aerosil), and sugars (glucose, fructose) are used to enhance the viscosity of the dispersion medium. They are known as suspending agents.

- List of suspending agents alginates methylcellulose hydroxyethylcellulose carboxymethylcellulose sodium carboxymethylcellulose microcrystalline cellulose acacia, tragacanth, xanthan gum bentonite carbomer powdered cellulose gelatin.
- Surfactants decrease the interfacial tension between drug particles and liquid and thus liquid is penetrated in the pores of drug particle displacing air from them and thus ensures wetting.
- Ideal requirements of packaging material it should be inert. It should effectively preserve the product from light, air, and other contamination through shelf-life. It should be cheap. It should effectively deliver the product without any difficulty.

PRACTICE QUESTIONS
LONG ANSWER TYPE QUESTIONS

1. What are different types of emulsions? How we can determine the type of emulsion?
2. What are emulsion? Give their advantages and disadvantages.
3. Discuss in detail about various types of emulsion with suitable examples.
4. How multiple emulsion are prepared give their pharmaceutical application?
5. Write in brief about various test used to differentiate between various types of emulsion.
6. Discuss in detail about various theories of emulsification?
7. Write short notes on additives used in formulation of emulsion:
   a. Emulsifying agent
   b. Preservatives
   c. Anti oxidant
   d. Auxillary emulsifier
8. Give various methods of preparation of emulsion with suitable example.

9. Give various methods of detecting physical instability of emulsion.

10. Discuss in detail about various chemical instability occurring in emulsion.

11. What are biphasic liquid dosage forms? Compare and contrast between suspension and emulsion.

12. What are different types of phases in suspension? Give advantages and disadvantages of suspension.

13. What are important factors which is to be kept in mind while formulating a suspension? Give pharmaceutical application of suspension.

14. Discuss in brief about various theories of suspension? Compare and contrast between flocculated and deflocculated suspension?

15. Write short notes on:
    a. Brownian movement
    b. Zeta potential
    c. Flocculating agent

16. Discuss in brief about quality control methods, packaging and labelling of suspension?

OBJECTIVE TYPE QUESTIONS

1. Which of the following is false regarding preservative:
   a. Effective against broad-spectrum of microorganisms
   b. Stable for its shelf-life
   c. Should be highly toxic
   d. Should not affect the stability of the active ingredient
   e. Free of taste and odour

2. When the two phases are immiscible like oil and water they form .... and then two phases are different like one is solid and other is liquid they form ....

3. In o/w emulsion, ... is in disperse phase whereas .... is in continuous phase.

4. Emulsifying agents reduce .... between two phases.

5. Emulsions meant for external use should be .... type.

6. Soaps formed from monovalent base produce .... emulsion and soaps from divalent base produce .... emulsion.

7. Bottle method is used for preparation of emulsions of .... and .... oils.

8. Match the following:

S. No	Type of water	Specification
1.	Potable water	A. Water prepared by distillation, by ion exchange resin method, or by reverse osmosis
2.	Purified water	B. Safe drinking water
3.	Aromatic waters	C. Clear saturated solutions of volatile oils, or other aromatic or volatile substances
4.	Sterile water	D. Free from microbes

9. Match the following:

S.No	Type of agents	Example/functions
1.	Buffering agents	A. Improve palatability and ease pourability of the product
2.	Isotonicity modifiers	B. 0.9% NaCl solution
3.	Viscosity modifiers	C. Propyl paraben
4.	Solubilizing agents	D. Resist the change in pH
5.	Preservatives	E. Enhances the solubility of the active ingredient in the solvent

10. Match the following

S.No	Type of agents	Example
1.	Antioxidants	A. Raspberry and ginger
2.	Sweetening agents	B. BHA, BHT
3.	Flavours	C. Carotenoids, chlorophylls
4.	Colouring agents	D. Aspartame

11. The particle size of the suspended drug particles in the suspension should be in the range of .... to .... micron.

12. The suspensions which are instilled into the eye should be free from .... particles.

13. The fine particle size of solid in suspension give a .... rate of ....

14. The particles form .... and from a .... like structure in case of flocculated suspension.

15. The flocculating agent reduces the .... and improved the .... of sold particles.

16. In non-flocculated suspension, the particle exists as ....

Answers

1. c
2. Emulsion, suspension
3. Oil, water
4. Interfacial tension
5. O/w type
6. O/w, w/o
7. Volatile, non-viscous
8. 1. B, 2. A, 3. C, 4. D
9. 1. D, 2. B, 3. A, 4. E, 5. C
10. 1. B, 2. D, 3. A, 4. C
11. 0.5, 5 micron
12. Gritty
13. Faster, dissolution
14. Loose aggregated, net work
15. Surface tension, dispersion
16. Separate entities

Chapter 7

Semisolid Dosage Forms

DEFINITION

Semisolid preparation are neither solid nor liquid formulation, they are dermatological preparations intended to apply externally on the skin to produce local or systemic effect. Semisolids adhere to the application surface for sufficiently long periods before they are washed off. This property helps prolong drug delivery at the application site. A semisolid dosage form is advantageous in terms of its easy application, rapid formulation, and ability to topically deliver a wide variety of drug substances (Flowchart 7.1).

Types of conventional semisolid dosage forms and their properties

Conventional semisolid dosage form mainly includes ointments, creams, pastes, gels or jellies, etc. A brief introduction about these is given in Table 7.1.

Ideal properties of semisolid dosage forms

  i. Smooth texture and elegant in appearance
 ii. Non dehydrating and non gritty
iii. Non greasy and non staining
 iv. Non hygroscopic and non irritating
  v. Do not alter membrane/skin functioning
 vi. Miscible with skin secretion.

Mechanisms of drug penetration and route of absorption

Skin anatomy: Semisolid dosage forms are generally used for topical administration of drugs. To understand the

Flowchart 7.1: Showing various semisolid dosage form

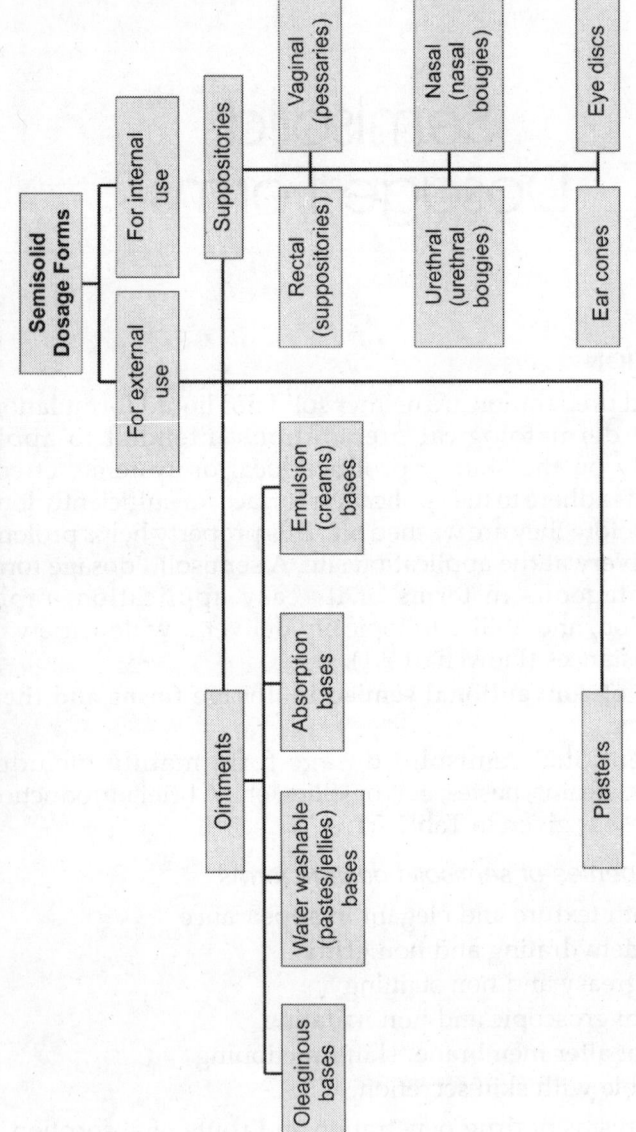

Table 7.1: A brief introduction of semisolid dosage forms

Dosage form	Properties
Ointments	• Ointments are soft semisolid preparations meant for external application to the skin or mucous membrane. • They usually contains medicament which is either dissolved or suspended in the base. • They have emollient and protective action.
Creams	• Creams are semisolid emulsions and are generally of softer consistency and lighter than ointments. • They are less greasy and are easy to apply.
Pastes	• Pastes are semisolid preparations for external application that differ from similar products in containing a high proportion of finely powdered medicaments. • They are stiffer and are usually employed for their protective action and for their ability to absorb serous discharges from skin lesions. • Thus when protective, rather than therapeutic action is desired, the formulation pharmacists will favour a paste, but when therapeutic action is required, he will prefer ointments and creams.
Jellies	• Jellies are transparent or translucent, non-greasy, semisolid preparation mainly used externally. • The gelling agent may be gelatin, starch, tragacanth, sodium alginate or cellulose derivative (e.g. carboxy methyl cellulose).

mechanism of drug penetration, the anatomy of skin should be known. The skin is made up of several layers including stratum corneum, viable epidermis and dermis, and it contains appendages that include sweat glands, sebaceous glands, and hair follicles. The stratum corneum is the outermost desquamating 'horny' layer of skin, comprising about 15–20 rows of flat, partially desiccated, dead, keratinized epidermal cells (Fig. 7.1)

Semisolid dosage forms for dermatological drug therapy are intended to produce desired therapeutic action at specific sites in the epidermal tissue. A drug's ability to penetrate the skin's

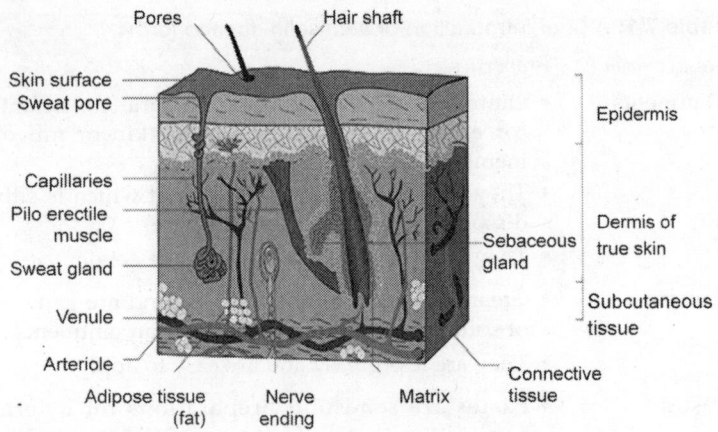

Fig. 7.1: Anatomy of cross-section of skin

epidermis, dermis, and subcutaneous fat layers depends on the properties of the drug (physicochemical properties), the carrier base and skin condition.

When a drug system is applied topically, the drug diffuses out of its vehicle onto the surface tissue of the skin. There are three potential portals of entry:

i. Through the follicular region

ii. Through the sweat ducts

iii. Through the unbroken stratum corneum between these appendages.

Absorption by the transdermal route, penetration is fairly rapid, although slower than intestinal tract absorption, and is almost always accompanied by some degree of pilosebaceous penetration as well.

Mechanism of Drug Absorption

Generally, drug absorption into the skin occurs by passive diffusion. The rate of drug transport across the stratum corneum follows Fick's Law of Diffusion,

According to Fick's Law

$$dA/dt = D.\Delta C.K/h$$

where

dA/dt is the steady-state flux across stratum corneum

D is the diffusion coefficient or diffusivity of drug molecules

ΔC is the drug concentration gradient across the stratum corneum

K is the partition coefficient of the drug between skin and formulation medium

h is the thickness of the stratum corneum.

Diffusion through the horny layer is a passive process. The passive process is affected only by the substance being absorbed, by the medium in which the substance is dispersed and by ambient conditions. Transport of lipophilic drug molecules is facilitated by their dissolution into intercellular lipids around the cells of the stratum corneum. Absorption of hydrophilic molecules into skin can occur through pores or openings of the hair follicles and sebaceous glands, but the relative surface area of these openings is barely 1% of the total skin surface. This small surface area limits the amount of drug absorption.

Factors Affecting Skin Penetration

The factors that influence skin penetration are the rate of diffusion depending primarily on the physicochemical property of drug like vehicle, pH, and concentration. The temperature of skin and the concentration of the drug play significant roles, but they are secondary to that of hydration.

The solubility of a drug determines the concentration presented to the absorption site, the water or lipid partition coefficient influences the rate of transport. An inverse relationship appears to exist between the absorption rate and the molecular weight. Small molecules penetrate more rapidly than large molecules, but within a narrow range of molecular size, there is little correlation between the size and the penetration rate.

OINTMENTS

Ointments are semisolid preparations for external application to skin or mucous membranes. The components of an ointment soften but do not melt upon application to the skin. Ointments

Pharmaceutics II

are used topically on a variety of body surfaces. These include the skin and the mucous membranes of the eye (an *eye ointment*), vagina, anus, and nose. An ointment may or may not be medicated. Therapeutically, ointments function as skin protective and emollients, but they are used primarily as vehicles for the topical application of drug substances. Since, they are greasy nature so they stain cloths. Ointments are usually very moisturizing, and good for dry skin, have low risk of sensitization because of having a few ingredients.

Characteristics of an Ideal Ointment

1. It should be chemically and physically stable.
2. It should be smooth and free from grittiness.
3. It should melt or soften at body temperature and be easily applied.
4. The base should be non-irritant and should have no therapeutic action.
5. The medicament should be finely divided and uniformly distributed throughout the base.

Classification of Ointments

Ointment can be classified into three types according to their therapeutic properties based on penetration of skin as follows (Table 7.2).

Table 7.2: Classification of ointment based on penetration of skin

(a) Epidermic ointments	*(b) Endodermic ointments*	*(c) Diadermic ointments*
• These ointments are intended to produce their action on the surface of the skin and produce local effect. • They are not absorbed • They act as protective, antiseptic and parasiticide.	• These ointments are intended to release the medicaments that penetrate into the skin. • They are partially absorbed and acts as emollients, stimulants and local irritants.	• These ointments are intended to release the medicaments that pass through the skin and produce systemic effects.

Methods of Preparation of Ointment

A well-prepared ointment should be:

a. Uniform throughout, i.e. it contains no lumps of separated high melting point ingredients of the base.

b. Free from grittiness, i.e. insoluble powders are finely subdivided and large lumps of particles are absent.

Ointments are prepared by following methods:

i. Fusion method
ii. Trituration method
iii. By chemical reaction
iv. By emulsification.

Ointments Prepared by Fusion method

When an ointment base contains a number of solid ingredients, such as white beeswax, cetyl alcohol, stearyl alcohol, stearic acid, hard paraffin, etc. as components of the base, it is required to melt them. The melting can be done in two methods:

Method I

The components are melted in the decreasing order of their melting point, i.e. the higher melting point substance should be melted first, the substances with next melting point and so on. The medicament is added slowly in the melted ingredients and stirred thoroughly until the mass cools down and homogeneous product is formed. This will avoid overheating of substances having low melting point.

Method II

All the components are taken in subdivided state and melted together. The maximum temperature reached is lower than Method I, and less time was taken possibly due to the solvent action of the lower melting point substances on the rest of the ingredients. Example is simple ointment BP.

Simple ointment BP

Wool fat	50 g
Hard paraffin	50 g
Cetostearyl alcohol	50 g
White soft paraffin	850 g

Method of Preparation

Hard paraffin and cetostearyl alcohol are mixed and heated on water bath. Wool fat and white soft paraffin are mixed and stirred until all the ingredients are melted. Allow it to cool and packed in suitable container.

Ointment Prepared by Trituration

This method is applicable when the base or a liquid is present in small amount.

i. Solids are finely powdered and passed through sieve.
ii. The powder is taken on an ointment-slab and triturated with a small amount of the base. To this additional quantities of the base are incorporated and triturated until the medicament is mixed with the base.
iii. Finally liquid ingredients are incorporated and mixed well, e.g.

Whitfield ointment (compound benzoic acid ointment BPC.)

Benzoic acid (fine powder)	6 g
Salicylic acid (fine powder)	3 g
Emulsifying ointment	91 g

Method: Benzoic acid and salicylic acid are sieved through sieve. They are mixed on the tile with small amount of base and mixed well until smooth paste is formed and finally make up the volume and dispensed.

Ointment Preparation by Chemical Reaction

Chemical reactions were involved in the preparation of several ointments for, e.g. non-staining iodine ointment BPC.

Iodine ointment, non-staining BPC

Iodine	5 g
Arachis oil	15 g
Yellow soft paraffin q.s.	100 g

i. Iodine is powdered and shaken with arachis oil at room temperature until dissolved and the temperature of the solution is raised to 50°C, with stirring until the brown colour disappears.

ii. Sufficient amount of yellow soft paraffin, heated to 40°C, poured into the iodine solution. Mixed well and kept in a wide-mouthed ointment jar and left undisturbed to cool down.

Preparation of Ointments by Emulsification

An emulsion system contains an oil phase, an aqueous phase and an emulsifying agent.

Example is cold cream

Sl. No.	Ingredients	Quantity
1.	Bees wax	80 g
2.	Mineral oil	490 ml
3.	Soft paraffin	70 g
4.	Cetyl alcohol	10 g
5.	Borax	4 g
6.	Perfume	Adequate
7.	Water q.s	1000 ml

Procedure: Take beeswax, soft paraffin, cetyl alcohol and mineral oil in a clean dry vessel and heat on water bath to 80°C. Dissolve borax in water in another vessel and heat simultaneously with the oil phase to 70°C. Add the aqueous phase to oil phase slowly with rapid stirring. Continue stirring slowly after the additions of aqueous phase until the cream has cooled to about 50°C. Add the perfume, mix well. Transfer it to a suitable container label it and dispense it.

PASTES

Pastes are the semisolid preparation meant for external application to the skin. They contain large amount of finely powdered solids like starch, zinc oxide, etc. Due to presence of these substances they have viscosity and stiffness and less attractive cosmetically. Since pastes are stiff they do not melt at ordinary temperature thus forming and holding a protective coating over the area they are applied.

Preparation of paste: They are prepared by trituration and fusion methods, trituration method is used when the base is liquid or semisolid while fusion method is used when the base is semisolid or solid in nature. Paste can be applied to the affected part with the help of a spatula or they may be spread on any of dressing material and then applied. They are not removed from the site of application for quite a long-time, the paste are not suitable for application to the scalp because they are very difficult to remove from the hair. Bases used for paste are:

1. Hydrocarbon bases
2. Water miscible bases
3. Water soluble bases

Hydrocarbon bases: Soft paraffin's and liquid paraffin are commonly used bases for the preparation of pastes.

Example: Prepare and dispense 1000 g of compound zinc paste BPC.

R_x

Zinc oxide, finely sifted	250 g
Starch, finely sifted	250 g
White, soft paraffin	500 g (qs)
Make a paste	

Method of preparation: Melt the white soft paraffin on a water bath. Separately pass the zinc oxide and starch through sieve no 120. Mix the required weight of powder in a warm mortar. Add small amount of melted base, with continuous trituration until smooth paste is obtained. Add the remaining part of the base mix until cold and uniform paste is obtained.

Example: Prepare and dispense 1000 g of aluminum paste, compound BPC.

R_x

Aluminium powder	200 g
Zinc oxide	400 g
Liquid paraffin	400 g (qs)
Make a paste	

Method: Mix aluminum powder and zinc oxide in a mortar. Add liquid paraffin with trituration thoroughly until smooth paste is obtained.

Water miscible bases: Emulsifying ointment is used as a water miscible base for the preparation of pastes. Similarly glycerin is also used as water miscible base for the preparation of pastes.

Example: Prepare and dispense 500 g of resorcinol and sulphur paste BPC.

R_x

Resorcinol, finely sifted	25 g
Precipitated sulphur	25 g
Zinc oxide, finely sifted	200 g
Emulsifying ointment	250 g
Make a paste	

Method of preparation: Triturate the zinc oxide, the resorcinol and precipitated sulphur with a portion of the emulsifying ointment until smooth and gradually incorporate the remaining part of the emulsifying ointment.

Water soluble bases: Suitable combination of high and low molecular weight polyethylene glycols are mixed together to get product of desired consistency which soften or melt when applied to the skin. These bases are water soluble. Water soluble dental paste containing neomycin sulphate is prepared with macrogol base.

Storage of pastes: The pastes should be stored in a well-closed container and in a cool place so as to prevent evaporation of moisture present in the paste. The difference between paste and ointment is given in Table 7.3.

GELS (JELLIES)

Gels are semisolid system in which a liquid phase is imbedded within a 3-D polymeric matrix (consisting of natural or synthetic gum) having a high degree of physical or chemical cross-linking or in other words gels are semisolid systems that consist of either suspensions of small inorganic particles or large organic molecules interpenetrated by a liquid. Gels can be either water based (aqueous gels) or organic solvent based (organogels).

Jellies are transparent or translucent non-greasy semisolid gels. Some are as transparent as water itself, an aesthetically pleasing state, other are turbid, as the polymer is present in colloidal aggregates that disperse light. They are used for medication, lubrication and some miscellaneous applications like carrier for spermicidal agents to be used intravaginally with diaphragms as an adjunctive means of contraception.

Table 7.3: Difference between pastes and ointments

Pastes	Ointments
1. They contain large amount of finely powdered solids, such as starch, zinc oxide, calcium carbonate, etc.	1. They contain medicaments which are generally dissolved/suspended/emulsified in the base
2. They are very thick and stiff	2. They are soft semisolid preparations
3. They are less greasy	3. They are more greasy
4. They are generally applied with a spatula or spread on lint	4. They are simply applied on the skin
5. They form a protective coating to the area where it is applied	5. They are used as protective or emollient for the skin
6. Paste contains a large amount of powder which is porous in nature, hence perspiration can escape	6. They are used for the protection of lesions
7. They are less macerating than ointments	7. They are more macerating in action

Types of Jellies

Medicated Jellies

Water soluble drugs like local anaesthetics, spermicides and antiseptics are suitable for incorporation in the jellies. They are easy to apply and evaporation of the water content produces a pleasant cooling effect. The medicinal film usually adheres well and gives protection but is easily removed by washing when the treatment is complete. Example is ephedrine sulfate jelly-used to arrest bleeding from nose.

Lubricant Jellies

Catheters, items of eletrodiagnostic equipment, such as cystoscopes, and rubber gloves or finger stalls used for rectal and other examinations require lubrication before use. (The lubricants must be sterile for articles inserted into sterile regions of the body, such as urinary bladder.

Miscellaneous Jellies

The following are more specialized jellies:

a. **Patch testing:** Here the jelly is the vehicle for allergens applied to the skin to detect sensitivity. Several allergens may be applied on one person. The viscosity of the jelly and it leaves on drying help to keep the particles separate.

b. **Electrocardiography:** To reduce electrical resistance between the patient's skin and electrodes of the cardiograph, an electrode jelly may be applied. This contains NaCl to provide good conductivity and often pumice powder which, when applied onto the skin, removes part of the horny layer of the epidermis, the main layer of electrical resistance.

Method of Preparation

Pharmaceutical jellies are usually prepared by adding a thickening agent such as tragacanth or carboxy methylcellulose (CMC) to an aqueous solution in which drug has been dissolved.

The mass is triturated in a mortar until a uniform product is obtained. For the preparation of jellies whole gum is preferred rather than powdered gum because the former gives a clear preparation of uniform consistency.

Formula

Ichthamol	1.0 g
Tragacanth	2.5 g
Alcohol 90%	5.0 g
Glycerin	1.0 g
Purified water q.s.	50.0 g

Procedure

i. Alcohol is taken in a 100 ml, wide mouthed jar; and then tragacanth is added to it. Mix it well.

ii. Water is added as quickly as possible and mixed.

iii. Separately ichthamol, glycerin and 10 ml water is mixed. Final weight is adjusted by adding more of water.

Preservation of Jellies

Since all the jellies contain large amount of water, therefore must be suitably preserved, e.g. methyl paraben 0.1 to 0.2% is commonly used. Bases and medicaments sensitive to heavy metals are sometimes protected by a chelating agent, e.g. ethylene diamine tetra acetic acid (EDTA).

Excipients Used in Preparation of Semisolids (Table 7.4)

Excipients used for formulating semisolids include API, Bases, antimicrobial preservative, chelating agents, humectants, fragrances.

Active Pharmaceutical Ingredients

Table 7.4: Medicaments prescribed for semisolids

Disease treated	API
Keratolytic	Salicylic acid
Acne	Sulphur, resorcinol
Antipruritic	Benzocaine, menthol, camphor
Emollient	Lanolin
Anti-inflammatory	Corticosteroid
Antifungal	Benzoic acid, salicylic acid

Bases

The base should be compatible with skin, stable, smooth and pliable, non-irritating, non-sensitizing, inert, capable of absorbing water or other liquid preparations, and of releasing the incorporated medicament, readily. A base for ophthalmic ointments must be non-irritating to the eye, should permit the diffusion of the drug through the secretions batting the eye, and should retain the activity of the medicament for a reasonable period often under proper storage conditions. It should also be sterilizable conveniently.

Selection of base depends on following:

1. Desired release rate of the drug substance from the base.
2. Rate and extent of topical drug absorption.
3. Desirability of occlusion of moisture from skin.
4. Stability of the drug in the ointment base.
5. Easy removal of base on washing.

Bases may be classified in several ways but the following classification based on composition is generally used which are as follow:

1. Oleaginous bases.
2. Absorption bases.
3. Emulsion bases.
4. Water soluble bases.
5. Water removable bases.

Oleaginous bases: These generally consist of a combination of more than one oleaginous material such as water-insoluble hydrophobic oils and fats. Most of the early ointment bases used to be exclusively oleaginous in nature but nowadays the materials obtained from plant, animal, mineral as well as synthetic origin is employed as oleaginous ointment bases. Combinations of these materials can produce a wide range of melting points and viscosities.

Absorption (emulsifiable) bases: These are essentially anhydrous systems composed of hydrophobic ingredients already discussed under oleaginous bases. They are called emulsifiable bases because they initially contain no water but are capable of taking it up to yield w/o and o/w emulsions. Absorption bases are w/o type emulsions and have capacity to absorb considerable quantities of water or aqueous solution without marked changes in consistency. Absorption bases are mostly mixtures of animal sterols with petrolatum. Combinations of cholesterol and/or other suitable lanolin fractions with white petrolatum are available under different commercial names, e.g. Eucerin and Aquaphor.

Emulsion bases: According to the type of emulsion, these bases are classified as either w/o or o/w. All w/o emulsions are not water-washable as the oil is in the external phase and o/w emulsions are used in dermatological preparations and cosmetic creams. Some of the popular creams include cold creams, vanishing creams. Skin creams, emollient creams, foundation creams, hand creams.

Water soluble bases: These include both anhydrous and hydrous dermatological non-emulsion bases which are water soluble and contain no oil phase. These are generally based on either polyethylene glycols or one or more of the other hydrocolloids.

Polyethylene glycols (carbowaxes) are water soluble, non-volatile, unctuous compounds. They do not hydrolyse or deteriorate and do not support mold growth. They have low irritancy and dermal/oral toxicities. Carbowaxes also allow easy diffusion of medicaments to the body tissues but the degree of their absorption is low. Different grade of cabowaxes are available which are designated by a number roughly representing their average molecular weights, e.g. 200, 300, 400, 600, 1000, 1540, 4000 and 6000. At room temperature, carbowaxes 200 to 400 are clear liquids whereas carbowaxes 1000 to 60,000 are white, waxy solids.

A variety of water washable ointment bases with consistencies ranging from semisolid to solid can be obtained by blending different polyethylene glycols. Polyethylene glycol ointment USP is a blend of carbowaxes 4000 and 400. Medicaments containing acidic hydrogen may interact with high molecular weight polyethylene glycols forming molecular complexes.

An example of formulation containing plastibase official in BPC is triamcinclone dental paste which contain an anti-inflammatory agent. Triamcinclone acetonide in adhesive, sodium CMC, pectin and gelatin.

Water removable bases: Popular example of this includes vanishing cream.

Note: Mineral oils are added to petrolatum to lower its fusion point, however by doing so problem of phase separation on storage is seen. This separation can be prevented by the addition of small quantities of natural waxes like ozokerite, ceresine or microcrystalline wax.

Semisolid ophthalmic vehicles contain soft petrolatum, a bland absorbing base or a water soluble base.

Antimicrobial Preservatives

Some base, although, resist microbial attack but because of their high water content, it require an antimicrobial preservative. Commonly used preservatives include methyl hydroxyl benzoate, propyl-hydroxybenzoate, chlorocresol, benzoic acid, phenyl mercuric nitrate, benzalkonium chloride, chlorhexidine acetate, benzyl alcohol and mercurial.

Antioxidants

An antioxidant is a molecule that inhibits the oxidation of other molecules. Oxidation is a chemical reaction that transfers electrons or hydrogen from a substance to an oxidizing agent. Oxidation reactions can produce free radicals. In turn, these radicals can start chain reactions. Antioxidants terminate these chain reactions by removing free radical intermediates, and inhibit other oxidation reactions. They do this by being oxidized themselves, so antioxidants are often reducing. Example of commonly used antioxidants includes butylated hydroxy anisole, butylated hydroxy toluene.

Chelating Agents

Chelating agents are chemical substances that contain molecules capable of bonding securely to minute particles of metal called ions. Example of commonly used chelating agents include citric acid, maleic acid, EDTA.

Humectants

A substance, especially a skin lotion used to reduce the loss of moisture example of commonly used humectants includes poly ethylene glycol, glycerol or sorbitol is added as humectants.

Fragrances

To impart fragrance to the formulation. Examples of widely use fragrances are lavender oil, rose oil, lemon oil, almond oil.

Emulsifier

Ideal properties of emulsifier includes:

a. Must reduce surface tension for proper emulsification (Tables 7.5 and 7.6).
b. Prevents coalescence should quickly absorb around the dispersed phase.
c. Ability to increase the viscosity at low concentration.
d. Effective at low concentration.

Table 7.5: Emulsifiers

Anionic	Cationic	Nonionic
Alkyl sulfates	Quaternary	Polyoxyethylene alkyl-aryl
Soaps	ammonium	ethers
Dodecyl benzene	compounds	Polyoxyethylene fatty acid
sulfonate	Alkoxyalkylamines	ester
Lactylates		Polyoxyethylene sorbitan
Sulfosuccinates		esters
Monoglyceride		Sorbitan fatty acid esters
sulfonates		Glyceryl fatty acid esters
Phosphate ester		Sucrose fatty acid esters
Silicones		Polyoxyethylene-
Taurates		polyoxypropylene block
		polymers

Table 7.6: HLB system

	Emulsifier HLB and its application
HLB range	Application
4–6	W/o emulsifier
7–9	Wetting agent
8–18	O/w emulsifier
13–15	Detergent
10–18	Solubilizers

Gelling agents

These are organic hydrocolloids or hydrophilic inorganic substances. They are tragacanth, sodium alginate, pectin, starch, gelatin, cellulose derivatives, carbomer, and polyvinyl alcohol clays.

There are numerous gelling agents varying in gelling ability. Commonly used gelling agents are listed in Table 7.7.

Permeability Enhancer

Skin can act as a barrier and prevent deep penetration of drug molecules. With the introduction of various penetration enhancers, however, systemic drug delivery through the transdermal route has gained major footing (Tables 7.7 and 7.8).

Table 7.7: Gelling agents

Material	%	Brookfield viscosity 'CPS'
Carbomer 941 resin NF	0.15	2900
Carbomer 941 resin NF	0.25	6300
Carbomer 941 resin NF	0.50	44000
Carbomer 941 resin NF	1.00	81000
Sodium carboxymethyl cellulose	1.50	5000
Guar gum	1.50	8040
Methyl cellulose	2.00	5200
Locust bean gum	2.50	22800
Sodium alginate	2.50	10400

Table 7.8: Penetration enhancer used with drugs for topical semisolids

Sr. no	Permeation enhancer	Drugs used
1.	Menthol, carvacrol, linalool	Propranolol hydrochloride
2.	Limonene	Indomethacin, ketoprofen
3.	Geraniol, nerolidol	Diclofenac sodium
4.	Oleic acid	Piroxicam
5.	Lecithin	Hydrocortisone acetate, heparin
6.	Propylene-glycol-dipelargonate	Heparin

PACKAGING OF SEMISOLIDS

Most semisolid products are manufacture by heating and are filled into the container while cooling still in the liquid state. It is important to established optimum pour point, the best temperature for filling and set or congealing point, the temperature at which the product become immobile in the container.

Topical dermatological products are packed in either jar or tubes whereas ophthalmic, nasal, vaginal and rectal semisolid products are almost always packed in tubes.

All drug product containers and closures must be approved by stability testing of product in the final container in which it is marketed. This includes stability testing of filled container at room temperature, e.g. 20°C as well as under accelerated stability testing condition, e.g. 40–50°C.

Ointment jars are made up of clear or opaque glass or plastic. Some are coloured green, amber or blue. Opaque jars are used for light sensitive products, are porcelain white, dark green or amber.

When the ointment is use for ophthalmic, rectal, vaginal or nasal application, they are packed with special applicator tips.

Ointment, creams and gels are most frequently packed in 5, 15 and 30 g tubes. Ophthalmic ointments typically are packed in small aluminum or collapsible plastic tubes holding 3.5 g of ointment.

ISLOLATED KEY POINTS

- Semisolid dosage forms are dermatological preparations intended to apply externally on the skin to produce local or systemic effect.
- **Physical properties:** (a) Smooth texture, (b) Elegant in appearance, (c) Non dehydrating, (d) Non gritty, (e) Non greasy and non staining, (f) Non hygroscopic.
- **Physiological properties:** (a) Non irritating, (b) Do not alter membrane/skin functioning, (c) Miscible with skin secretion, (d) Have low sensitization effect.
- Ointments are semisolid preparations meant for external application to the skin or mucous membrane. They, usually contain a medicament or medicaments dissolves, suspended or emulsified in the base.
- Creams are viscous emulsions of semisolid consistency intended for application to the skin or mucous membrane two types o/w type w/o type.
- Pastes are the preparations contain a large amount of finely powdered solids, such as starch and zinc oxide. These are generally very thick and stiff.
- **Jellies:** These are thin transparent or translucent, non greasy preparations. They are similar to mucilages because they are prepared by using gums but they differ from mucilages in having jelly like consistency.
- **Gels:** These are jelly-like semisolid dispersions of drug meant to be applied on the skin.
- The skin is the largest organ of the body. Human skin is, on average, 0.5 mm thick (ranging from 0.05 mm in eyelid to 2 mm).

- **Skin structure:** The skin consists of three major layers: Epidermis dermis subcutaneous tissues.
- **Percutaneous absorption:** It involves passive diffusion of substance through skin. Transepidermal penetration: Intracellular penetration. Intercellular penetration. Transappendegeal penetration.
- **Bases:** There are four classes or types of bases which are differentiated on the basis of their physical composition. **These are:** Oleaginous bases. Absorption bases. Emulsifying base. (Water in oil emulsion bases and oil in water emulsion bases) and water soluble bases.
- **Selection of the appropriate base based on:** 1. Dermatological factors, 2. Pharmaceutical factors.
- **Methods of preparation of semisolids:** Trituration method fusion method emulsfication method: (a) preparation of oil and aqueous phases, (b) mixing of the phases, (c) cooling the emulsion, (d) homogenization, (4) chemical reaction method.
- **Trituration method:** It is the most commonly used for the preparation of semisolid. When base contains soft fats and oils, or medicament is insoluble or liquid, then this method is used with spatula or mortar and pestle.
- **Fusion method:** The ingredients of the base are melted together and properly mixed to obtain a uniform product. On small scale, fusion method is carried out in a porcelain dish, which is placed in a water bath.
- Emulsification method preparation of oil and aqueous phases place the ingredients of the oil phase into the stainless steel steam-jacketed kettle and melt them whilst mixing.

PRACTICE QUESTIONS
LONG ANSWER TYPE QUESTIONS

1. What are semisolid dosage forms? Discuss in brief about various types of semisolid dosage form along with their properties.
2. Discuss in brief about ideal properties of semisolid dosage form.
3. What are the various factors affecting drug penetration and route of absorption of semisolid dosage form?

4. Give mechanism of drug absorption in detail. How various types of skin structure govern mechanism of absorption?

5. What are ointments? Give classification and discuss in brief about ideal characteristics of an ointment.

6. What are the various ingredients used in the preparation of semisolid dosage form? Give suitable examples.

7. Write short notes on:
   a. Bases
   b. Preservatives
   c. Antioxidant
   d. Chelating agent
   e. Humectrants
   f. Surfactants

8. What are the various types of permeability enhancer? Give there mechanism of action.

9. Give various methods of preparation of ointments with suitable example.

10. What are pastes? Give properties of an ideal paste.

11. Compare and contrast between paste and ointment.

12. Discuss in detail about the various bases used in the preparation of pastes. Give methods of preparation of pastes.

13. Write short notes on:
    a. Gels
    b. Types of jellies
    c. Packaging of semisolid dosage forms.

14. What are the various evaluation methods used for evaluation of semisolid dosage form?

15. Write in brief about recent development in semisolid dosage form. What are the advantages and disadvantages of novel approach?

OBJECTIVE TYPE QUESTIONS

1. Semisolid dosage forms are dermatological preparations intended to apply........................ on the skin to produce local or systemic effect.

2. .... also known as cataplasms and are soft viscous wet masses of solid substances.
3. The skin consists of three major layers ....
4. The phase which is dispersed in a medium is known as an...

Answers

1. Externally
2. Poultices
3. Epidermis dermis subcutaneous tissues
4. Internal phase or dispersed phase

Chapter 8

Suppositories

INTRODUCTION

Suppositories are solid unit dosage forms suitable shaped for insertion into the rectum. The bases used either melt when warmed to body temperature, or dissolve or disperse when in contact with mucous secretions. Suppositories may contain medicaments which are intended to exert a systemic effect, either dissolved or dispersed in the base. Suppositories are prepared by incorporating any medicaments in the base, which may then be shaped by cold compression into moulds. The molten mass is poured at a suitable temperature into moulds and allowed to cool until set.

Pessaries are solid unit dosage forms suitably shaped for insertion into the vagina, and containing medicaments intended to exert a local action. They may be prepared by moulding as described above or may be compressed as suitably shaped tablets.

The ideal suppository base should be nontoxic, nonirritating, inert, compatible with medicaments, and easily formed by compression or molding. It should also dissolve or disintegrate in the presence of mucous secretions or melt at body temperature to allow for the release of the medication. The suppository base composition plays an important role in rate and extent of release of medications.

The shapes of suppositories are generally tapering at one end and depending upon the need various sizes are prepared (Fig. 8.1)

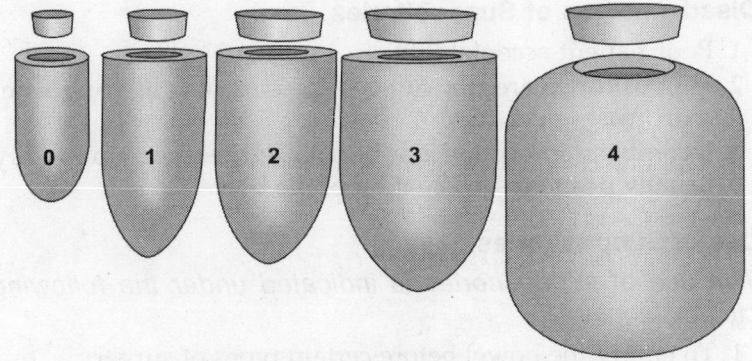

Fig. 8.1: Various types of suppositories

Number 0 is for children, and can also be used for the ear or nose.

Number 1, 2, and 3 are for the rectum, number 4 is a pessary.

Advantages of Suppositories

1. Suppositories are dosage forms containing accurate quantities of medicament(s).
2. When the oral administration is not suitable, as in unconscious patients and infants suppositories are used for systemic effect.
3. Suppositories allow administration of some medicaments, which are sensitive to the gastric pH and gastric enzymes and are not tolerated orally.
4. Suppositories permit administration of medicament that interrupt the functionality of the gastrointestinal tract, e.g. drugs irritating to the stomach. Also suitable in case of nausea and vomiting.
5. Drugs destroyed by first past metabolism in portal circulation may bypass the liver circulation, where many drugs are subject to metabolic changes (first pass effect).
6. Suppositories are suitable when local effect is wanted as in the treatment of rectal, vaginal and urethral diseases.
7. Suppositories have shown faster onset of action than found after oral administration as the drug is directly absorbed from the mucosa into the venous circulation.

Disadvantages of Suppositories

1. Poor patient acceptability.
2. Suppositories are not suitable for patients suffering from diarrhea.
3. Incomplete absorption may be obtained because suppository usually promotes evacuation of the bowel.

Use of Suppositories

The use of suppositories is indicated under the following circumstances:

1. To empty the bowel before certain types of surgery.
2. To empty the bowel to relieve acute constipation or when other treatments for constipation have failed.
3. To empty the bowel before endoscopic examination.
4. To introduce medication into the system.
5. To soothe and treat hemorrhoids or anal pruritus.

Routes of Administration that Utilize Suppositories

They are made in a variety of shapes and sizes because they are used in many different routes of administration (body cavities).

Rectal

Rectal route is used for local effect or to achieve a systemic effect. Local effects may include the soothing of inflamed hemorrhoidal tissues, promoting laxation, and enemas. Using rectal administration to achieve systemic activity is preferred when the drug is destroyed in the GI tract, if oral administration is not possible because of vomiting, or the patient is unconscious or incapable of swallowing oral formulations. Rectal administration has been used to treat a variety conditions, such as asthma, nausea, motion sickness, anxiety, and bacterial infections.

The most common rectal formulations are suppositories, solutions, and ointments. Suppositories are manufactured in a variety of shapes. Rectal suppositories for adults are tapered at one end and usually weigh about 2 g. Infant rectal suppositories usually weight about 1 g or about half that of adult suppositories.

The major disadvantages of rectal suppositories:
1. Poor patient acceptability; they are inconvenient.
2. Rectal absorption of most drugs is frequently erratic and unpredictable.
3. Some suppositories "leak" or are expelled after insertion.

Vaginal Suppositories

Vaginal administration has many advantages.
1. Generally, there is less drug degradation via this route of administration compared to oral administration
2. The dose can be retrieved if necessary
3. There is the potential of long-term drug absorption with various intrauterine devices (IUDs).

Vaginal administration does lead to variable absorption since, the vagina is a physiologically and anatomically dynamic organ that causes pH and membrane permeability to change over time. There is also a tendency of some dosage forms to be expelled after insertion into the vagina.

Vaginal formulations include solutions, powders for solutions, ointments, creams, aerosol foams, suppositories, and tablets. Vaginal suppositories are employed as contraceptives, feminine hygiene antiseptics, bacterial antibiotics, or to restore the vaginal mucosa. Vaginal suppositories are inserted high in the vaginal tract with the aid of a special applicator. The suppositories are usually globular, oviform, or cone-shaped and weigh between 3 and 5 g. Patients should be instructed to quickly dip the suppository in water before insertion. Because suppositories are generally used at bedtime and can be messy if the formulation is an oleaginous base, patients should wear a sanitary napkin to protect nightwear and bedlinens.

Urethral

Urethral suppositories are cylindrical in shape (3–6 mm in diameter) and vary in length according to gender. Female urethral suppositories can be 25–70 mm in length while male urethral suppositories can be about 50–125 mm in length. The one commercially available urethral suppository is actually marketed as a "pellet," and is 1.4 mm in diameter and 3 or 6 mm in length depending on strength. Urethral suppositories are unusual and may not be encountered in a compounding practice.

Inserting Suppositories

Inserting Rectal Suppositories (Fig. 8.2)

1. If possible, go to the toilet and empty bowels.
2. Wash hands carefully with soap and warm water.

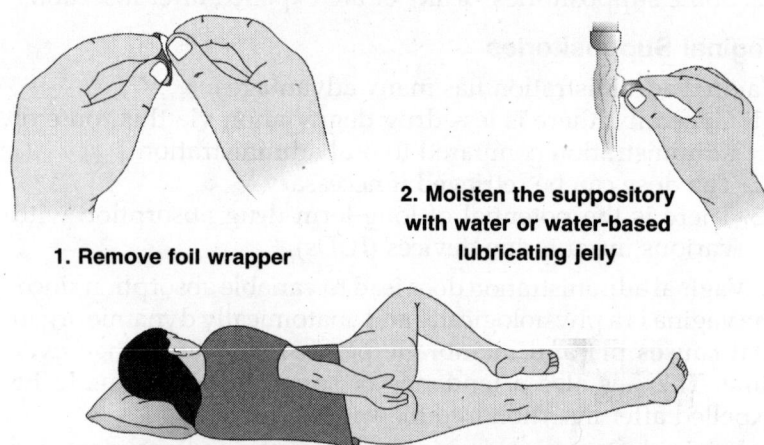

1. Remove foil wrapper

2. Moisten the suppository with water or water-based lubricating jelly

3. Lie on your left side and bend your right knee up toward your chest. Gently push the suppository into your rectum

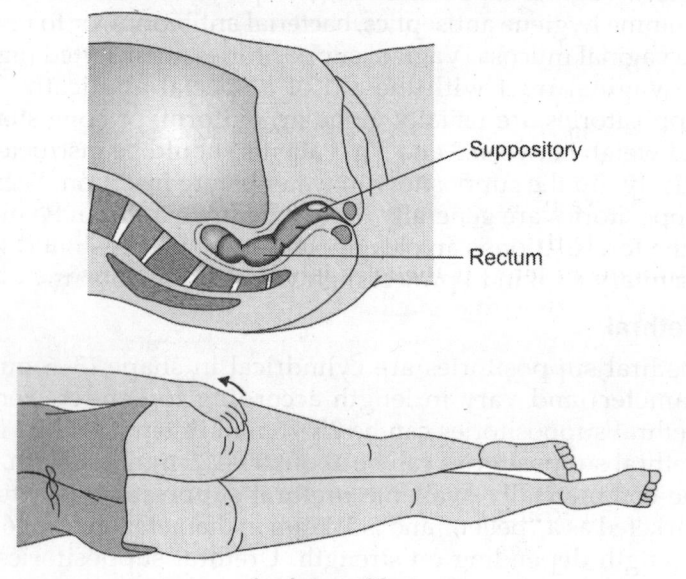

Suppository

Rectum

Laying position

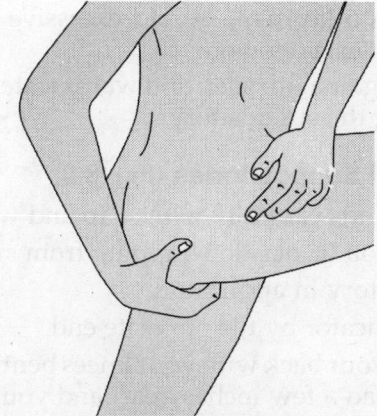

Standing position

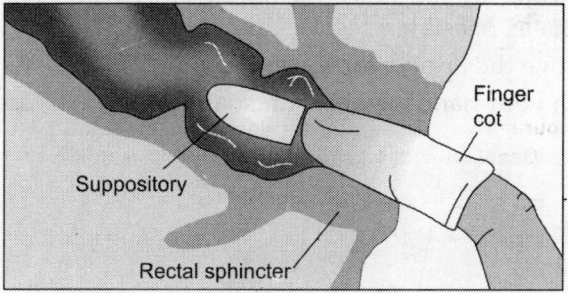

Fig. 8.2: Method of inserting rectal suppository

3. Remove any foil or plastic wrapping from the suppository.
4. Lubricate the tapered end of the suppository with a small amount of Jelly. If the jelly is not available, moisten the suppository with a small amount of water.
5. Either stand with one leg on a chair, or lay on one side with one leg straight and the other leg bent toward your stomach.
6. Separate buttocks to expose the rectal area.
7. Gently but firmly push the suppository into the rectum until it passes the sphincter (about 1/2 to 1 inch in infants, and 1 inch in adults.
8. Close your legs and sit (or lay) still for about 15 minutes. Avoid emptying bowels for at least one hour (unless the

suppository is a laxative). Avoid excessive movement or exercise for at least one hour.

9. Wash hands again with soap and warm water immediately after inserting the suppository.

Inserting Vaginal Suppositories (Fig. 8.3)

1. Wash your hands carefully with soap and warm water.
2. Remove any foil or plastic wrapping from suppository.
3. Place suppository in applicator.
4. Hold the applicator by the opposite end.
5. Either lay on your back with your knees bent, or stand with your feet spread a few inches apart and your knees bent.
6. Gently insert the applicator into the vagina as far as it will go comfortably. Once you are ready, push the inside of the applicator in and place the suppository as far back in the vagina as possible.
7. Remove the applicator for the vagina.
8. Wash your hands again with soap and warm water.

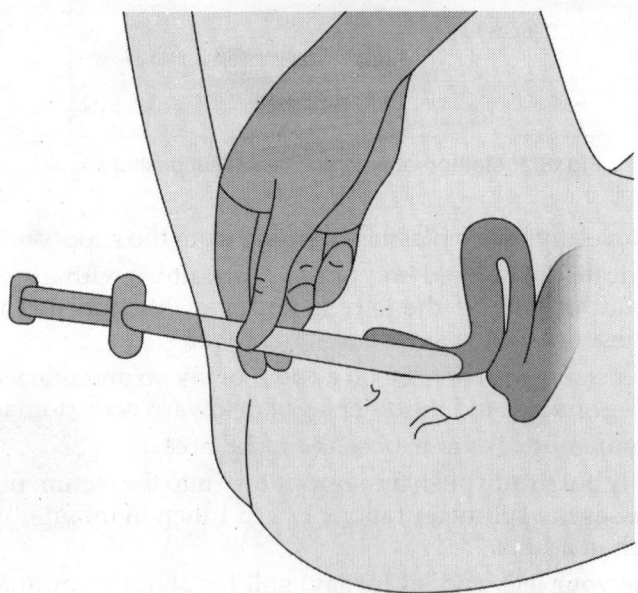

Fig. 8.3: Method of inserting vaginal suppository

Types of Suppository Bases
Four main types of bases are available:
1. Oily bases.
2. Hydrophilic bases.
3. Water dispersible bases.
4. Emulsifying bases.

Oily or Oleaginous or Fatty Bases
Cocoa Butter (Theobroma Oil)
One of the most widely used suppository base, used in compounding prescription when no base is specified. Cocoa butter is defined as the fat obtained from roasted seed of Theobroma cacao. Chemically, it is a triglyceride with the predominant glyceride chains being oleopalmitostearin and oleodistearin. It is a yellowish-white, solid, brittle fat, which smells and tastes like chocolate. Because cocoa butter can easily melt and rancidify, it must be stored in cool, dry place, and protected from light.

Advantages
1. Has a melting point range of 34–38°C. (i.e. solid at normal room temperature but melts at body temperature).
2. Readily melts on warming, rapid sets on cooling.
3. Easily miscible with other ingredients.
4. Bland, innocuous, non-reactive and non-irritating.

Disadvantages
1. Gets adhere to the mould: Sticking is a problem which may be overcome by adequate lubrication.
2. Softening point too low for hot climate.
3. Melting point reduced by soluble ingredients, additives, such as beeswax may be incorporated to raise the melting point sufficiently to counteract the effects of medicaments and/or climate.
4. Rancid on storage due to oxidation of unsaturated glycerides.
5. Poor water absorbing ability. Improved by the addition of emulsifying agents.

6. Leakage from the body. Sometimes melted base escape from the rectum or vagina, for this reason, oil of theobroma is rarely used as a pessary base.
7. It is costly.
8. Shows polymorphism.

Emulsified Theobroma oil

In order to increase the diffusion and absorption, several agents have been used to form emulsified theobroma oil suppositories. The addition of an emulsifying agent to cocoa butter also prevents unnecessary melting because the suppository will swell and disintegrate in the presence of moisture. Thus, the melting point may be raised without fear of interfering with disintegration. Also, more aqueous solution may be incorporated in such emulsified suppositories.

Examples: The addition of 5% glyceryl monostearate has been recommended for preparing emulsified cocoa butter suppositories. These products are said to have a melting point above 35°C and may be made by either the hot or the cold method.

The incorporation of 2 to 3% cetyl alcohol with theobroma oil also makes a satisfactory emulsified base. A suppository mass containing 2% lecithin and 98% theobroma oil forms an oil-in-water emulsified base. A water-in-oil emulsion is formed by the inclusion of 2% cholesterol with theobroma oil.

Synthetic Hard Fat (Hydrogenated Oils)

Synthetic hard fat bases are prepared by first hydrolyzing the vegetable oil, then hydrogenating the resulting fatty acids and finally reemulsifying the acids by heating with glycerol, e.g. hydrogenated palm kernel oil is used in tropical countries as a base for suppositories.

Hydrophilic Bases
Glycerinated Gelatin

This substance has many properties that make it a desirable base for suppositories. Suppositories made with glycerinated gelatin slowly dissolve in the aqueous secretions and provide a slow, continuous release of medication. Glycerinated gelatin may be used to prepare all types of suppositories and it is particularly useful in vaginal suppositories. It is well-adapted for the incorporation of solid extracts such as belladonna. It also may be used for suppositories containing boric acid; bromides, chloral hydrate, iodide, iodoform and other drugs. Care should be taken in the selection of the type of gelatin used in suppositories. There are two major types of gelatin, each of which has its specific applications.

Type A (also called pharmagel A) is derived from an acid-treated precursor and has a pH between 3.8 and 4.5. This gelatin has an isoelectric point between pH 7 and 9. In solution, type A gelatin carries a strong positive charge and behaves as a cationic agent. It has the customary incompatibilities of both a weak acid and chlorides.

Type B (also called pharmagel B). It is made from an alkali treated precursor and has a pH between 5 and 7. Since, this pH is above its isoelectric point (pH 4.7 to 5), it carries a negative charge and behaves as an anionic agent, unless its pH is lowered below 4.7, when it becomes cationic.

The type of gelatin selected must be based upon the properties of the medicament to be incorporated. It was found that ichthammol suppositories made with type A gelatin were granular. Mild silver protein suppositories made with type A gelatin shrink because they contain protein that is anionic in relation to the cationic properties of type A gelatin. Glycerinated gelatin is also the best and most reliable vehicle for the effective use of antiseptics, such as hexyl resorcinol, nitromersol, and phemerol in suppository form. Many formulae have been recommended for glycerinated gelatin, differing in the proportion of glycerin, gelatin, and water.

Advantages

1. The base does not melt at body temperature, but rather dissolve in the secretions of the cavity in which they are inserted.
2. Solution time is regulated by the proportion of gelatin: glycerin: water used, the nature of gelatin used, and the chemical reaction of the drug with gelatin.
3. The consistency of a 20% gelatin formula was found inadequate for rectal use. The gelatin content is sometimes increased to as high as 30%.

Disadvantages

1. Glycerol suppositories have laxative action.
2. Unpredictable solution time. This varies with the batch of gelatin and the age of the base.
3. The base requires protection from heat and moisture and also has a dehydrating effect on the rectal or vaginal mucosa leading to irritation.
4. The base may require preservatives leading to problems of incompatibility.
5. The base is more time consuming to prepare than fatty bases and may be difficult to remove from the mould.
6. Lubrication of the mould is essential.

The Polyethylene Glycols (Macrogols)

Polyethylene glycols are polymers of ethylene oxide and water, prepared to various chain length, molecular weights, and physical states. Polyglycols exist as liquids when their average molecular weight ranges from 200 to 600, and as wax-like solids with molecular weights about 1000. Their water solubility, hygroscopicity and vapor pressure decrease with increasing average molecular weights.

The polyethylene glycol suppositories can be prepared by both moldings and cold compression methods.

Several combinations of polyethylene glycols have been prepared for suppository bases having desired consistency and different physical characteristics.

Advantages

1. No laxative effect.
2. Microbial contamination less likely.
3. The base contracts slightly on cooling and no lubricant is necessary.
4. Melting point generally above body temperature. Cool storage is therefore not so critical; they are suitable for hot climates and less likely to melt on handling. The high melting point also means that the bases do not melt in the body but dissolve and disperse the medication slowly, providing a sustained effect.

5. Produce high viscosity solution. This means that after dispersing in the body, leakage is less likely.

6. Good solvent properties.

7. Give product with clean smooth appearance.

Disadvantages

1. **Hygroscopic:** Like glycerogelatin base, polyethylene glycol bases may cause irritation to the mucosa. This can partly overcome by incorporation of 20% water in the mass or by instructing the patient to dip the preparation in water prior to insertion.

2. **Poor bioavailability of medicaments:** The good solvent properties may result in retention of the drug in the liquefied base with consequence reduction in therapeutic effect.

3. **Incompatibilities:** Polyethylene glycol bases are incompatible with some medicaments, e.g. bismuth salts, ichthamol, benzocaine and phenol, and reduces the activity of quaternary ammonium compounds and hydroxybenzoate. They also interact with some plastics which limits the choice of container.

4. **Brittleness:** Polyethylene glycol suppositories may be brittle unless poured at as low temperature as possible. The addition of surface active agents or plasticizer may reduce brittleness. Products sometimes fracture on storage, particularly if they contain water. One cause is the high solubility of the macrogols, which can lead to a supersaturated solution in the water and subsequent crystallization. This in turn makes the mass granular and brittle.

5. Crystal growth of certain medicaments may occur, particularly if they are partly in solution or suspension in the base.

Soap Glycerin

Stearin soap (i.e. curd soap, sodium stearate) is used as a suppository base. The soap used in this base is formed in glycerin solution by interaction between stearic acid and sodium carbonate.

It has certain *advantages* over gelatin for making glycerin sufficiently hard for suppositories:

1. A larger quantity of glycerin can be incorporated actually up to 95% of the mass.
2. Soap assists the action of glycerin, whereas gelatin dose not.

The *disadvantage* is that soap glycerin suppositories are very hygroscopic, and require to be wrapped in waxed paper or pure tin foil, and protected from the atmosphere.

Water Dispersible Bases

Several non-ionic surfactants can be used for formulating both water-soluble and oil-soluble drugs. The water dispersible bases offer the additional advantages of storage and handling at elevated temperatures having broad drug compatibility, non support of microbial growth, non toxicity, and non sensitivity. The surfactants most commonly used in suppository formulations are the Tween, Myrj, Span and Ariacel. These surfactants may be used alone, blended or in combination with other suppository vehicle materials to yield a wide range of melting points and consistencies.

Emulsifying Bases

Massa Estrinum (Adeps Solidus)

This is a mixture of the monoglycerides, diglycerides, and triglycerides of the saturated fatty acids having the formula $C_{11}H_{23}COOH$ to $C_{17}H_{35}COOH$.

Several grades are available to suit climate changes, such as Massa estrinum A, AB, AS, B, BB, BC, BD and C. They possess a melting range of 33 to 38°C.

Massupol

This consists of glyceryl esters, mainly of lauric acid, to which a very small amount of glyceryl monostearate has been added. They exhibit a melting range of 34–37°C, and are suitable for mass production.

Witepsol

They consist of hydrogenated triglycerides of lauric acid with added monoglycerides. Nine grades are available of which

Witepsol H_{12}, H_{15}, W_{35}, S_{55}, E_{75} and E_{55} are in common uses. The fatty acids, of which the trigycerides in Witepsol are composed, are derived from natural saturated fatty acid of C_{12}–C_{18} with predominance of lauric acid. They are formerly marketed under the trade name of Imhausen bases. They are suitable for formulation of eutectic mixtures and tropical suppositories, e.g. Witepsol H_{15} disintegrates almost as fast in the rectum as cocoa butter. The melting times were 4 minutes for cocoa butter, 6 minutes for Witepsol.

Wecobee Bases

They are triglycerides of higher melting fractions of coconut oil and palm kemal oil and may contain 0.25% of lecithin. The incorporation of glyceryl monosterate and propylene glycol monostearate makes them emulsifiable. Wecobee W, R, S, M and FS are presented in commerce.

Dehydarz Bases

Three grades are manufactured and marketed as suppository base I, II and G. Base I and II are composed of hardened fatty alcohols and fats, but base G is formed from a saturated fatty alcohols known as Guerbet alcohols. Waxes or high-melting alcohol may be added to raise the melting point of base I and base II.

None of the Dehydag exhibits polymorphism. They may be heated above their melting points without lowering their congealing temperatures. Waxes or high melting alcohols may be added to raise the m.p. of these bases.

Emulsified Propylene Glycol Derivatives

Propylene glycol α-monostearate (monolene) was developed as a suppository base. This base melts within body temperature and it is self-emulsifying in water, forming soft bulky non-irritant emulsion, suitable for rectal treatment. Its properties permit diffusion of the medicament and absorption of water soluble drug irrespective of melting range, while insoluble substances are emulsified and kept in intimate contact with mucosal tissue.

Advantages of emulsifying bases

1. The physical properties do not change by overheating.
2. They do not stick to the mould.

3. They solidify rapidly.
4. As they all contain an emulsifying agent, they can absorb fairly high percentages of aqueous liquids.
5. The emulsifying agents are monoglycerides which form water-in-oil emulsions and this would seem more rational than the use of oil-in water emulsifying agents.

Methods of Preparation

Suppositories can be extemporaneously prepared by one of three methods.

Hand Rolling method

Hand rolling is the oldest and simplest method of suppository preparation and may be used when only a few suppositories are to be prepared in a cocoa butter base. It has the advantage of avoiding the necessity of heating the cocoa butter. A plastic-like mass is prepared by triturating grated cocoa butter and active ingredients in a mortar. The mass is formed into a ball in the palm of the hands, then rolled into a uniform cylinder with a large spatula or small flat board on a pill tile. The cylinder is then cut into the appropriate number of pieces which are rolled on one end to produce a conical shape.

Effective hand rolling requires considerable practice and skill. The suppository "pipe" or cylinder tends to crack or hollow in the center, especially when the mass is insufficiently kneaded and softened (Fig. 8.4).

a. Mix measured quantity of medicinal substances with sufficient quantity of theobroma oil.
b. Triturate and, if required, soften with diluted alcohol and rub until a smooth paste is formed.

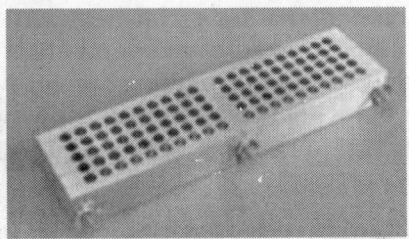

Fig. 8.4: Suppository hand mould

c. Add remaining quantity of theobroma oil and add wool fat for consistency.

d. When the mass becomes plastic by vigorous kneading of the pestle quickly remove from the mortar with a spatula.

e. Transfer with spatula to a piece of filter paper and keep in hands during the kneading and rolling procedure.

f. Roll the mass by quick rotating movements of the hands and immediately place on a pill tile.

g. Rolling the mass on the tile with a flat board forms a cylindrical suppository.

h. Cut in pieces by spatula (Fig. 8.5).

i. Give the shape by rolling one end on the tile with a spatula.

j. Pack in butter paper or in proper container and store in cool place.

Compression Mould Suppositories (Cold Compression)

Compression molding is a method of preparing suppositories from a mixed mass of grated suppository base and medicaments which is forced into a special compression mold. The method requires that the capacity of the molds first be determined by compressing a small amount of the base into the dies and weighing the finished suppositories. When active ingredients are added, it is necessary to omit a portion of the suppository base, based on the density factors of the active ingredients.

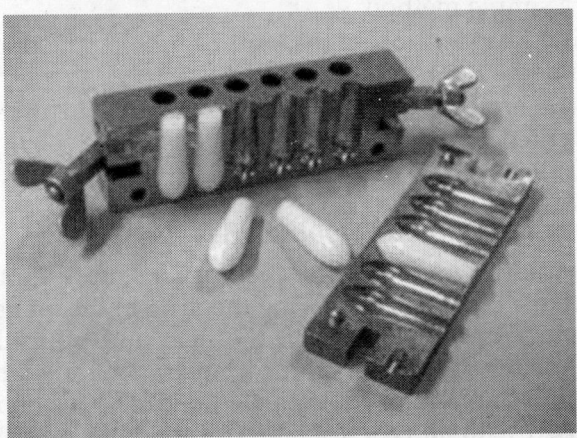

Fig. 8.5: Suppository hand mould (open)

The prepared mass C is placed in a cylinder A. It is forced through narrow opening D by means of piston B into a mould. Threads of mass pass in the mould G and are compressed until a homogenous fused mass is formed in E. On removal of retaining plate F the suppositories are ejected by further pressure (Fig. 8.6). The mass and compression cylinder of the machine may be chilled to prevent heat of compression from making the mass too fluid. Useful suppositories containing insoluble solids and thermolabile drugs. It is not suitable for glycero-gelatin products.

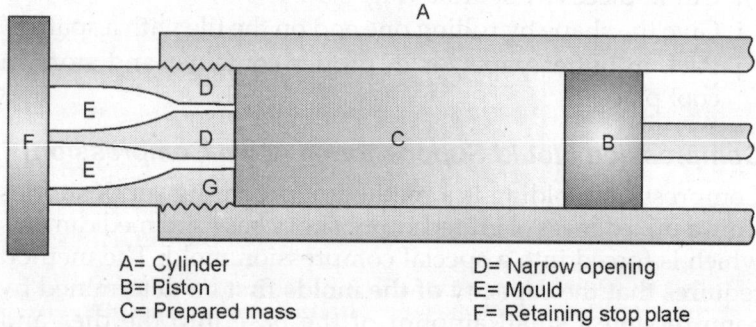

A= Cylinder   D= Narrow opening
B= Piston   E= Mould
C= Prepared mass   F= Retaining stop plate

Fig. 8.6: Cold compression machine for suppositories

The major Advantages of this process are:

1. It is a simple method
2. It gives suppositories that are more elegant than hand moulded suppositories
3. In this method sedimentation of solids in the base is prevented
4. Suitable for heat labile medicaments.

Fusion or Melt Mould Suppositories

Fusion molding involves first melting the suppository base, and then dispersing or dissolving the drug in the melted base. The mixture is removed from the heat and poured into a suppository mold. When the mixture has congealed, the suppositories are removed from the mold. The fusion method can be used with all types of suppositories and must be used with most of them.

Suppositories are generally made from solid ingredients and drugs which are measured by weight. When they are mixed, melted, and poured into suppository mold cavities, they occupy a volume—the volume of the mold cavity. Since, the components are measured by weight but compounded by volume, density calculations and mold calibrations are required to provide accurate doses.

Calibration of mould is necessary before preparing suppositories and pessaries. The capacity of the mould varies with the different bases. Each mould should be calibrated using the base alone, weighing the products and taking the mean weight as true capacity. When a drug is placed in a suppository base, it will displace an amount of base as a function of its density. If the drug has the same density as the base, it will displace an equivalent weight of the base. If the density of the drug is greater than that of the base, it will displace a proportionally smaller weight of the base. Density factors for common drugs in cocoa butter are available in standard reference texts. The density factor is used to determine how much of a base will be displaced by a drug. For example, aspirin has a density factor in cocoa butter of 1.3. If a suppository is to contain 0.3 g of aspirin, it will replace 0.3 g ÷ 1.3 or 0.23 g of cocoa butter. If the blank suppository (suppository without the drug) weighed 2 g, then g – 0.23 g or 1.77 g of cocoa butter will be needed for each suppository, and the suppository will weigh 1.77 g + 0.3 g = 2.07 g. So, if a pharmacist was making 12 aspirin suppositories using cocoa butter as the base, he would weigh 1.77 g × 12 or 21.24 g of cocoa butter and 0.3 g × 12 or 3.6 g of aspirin.

ISOLATED KEY POINTS

- Suppositories are medicated solid dosage forms of various shapes and sizes meant for insertion into body cavities like rectum, vagina, urethra, ear and nose.
- Suppositories are suited particularly for producing local action, but may also be used to produce a systemic effect or to exert a mechanical effect to facilitate emptying the lower bowel.
- Suppository Base; (1) Oleaginous (fatty) bases: Cocoa butter or Theobroma oil; (2) Water soluble or miscible bases: Glycerinated gelating, polyethylene glycol.

- Suppositories method of preparation: Hand rolling is the oldest and simplest method of suppository preparation and may be used when only a few suppositories are to be prepared in a cocoa butter base. A plastic-like mass is prepared by triturating grated cocoa butter and active ingredients in a mortar.
- Compression molding compression molding is a method of preparing suppositories from a mixed mass of grated suppository base and medicaments which is forced into a special compression mold using suppository making machines. The suppository base and the other ingredients are combined by thorough mixing. The friction of the process causing the base to soften into a past-like consistency.
- On a small scale, a mortar and pestle may be used (preheated mortar facilitate softening of the base). On large scale, mechanically operated kneading mixers and a warmed mixing vessel may be applied. In the compression machine, the suppository mass is placed into a cylinder which is then closed. Pressure is applied from one end to release the mass from the other end into the suppository mold or die.
- **Fusion molding involves:** (1) Melting the suppository base, (2) Dispersing or dissolving the drug in the melted base, (3) The mixture is removed from the heat and poured into a suppository mold, (4) Allowing the melt to congeal (5) Removing the formed suppositories from the mold. The fusion method can be used with all types of suppositories and must be used with most of them.
- Suppository molds small scale molds are capable of producing 6 or 12 suppositories in a single operation. Industrial molds produce thousands of suppositories per hour from a single molding.
- Packaging suppositories must be packed in such a manner that they do not touch each other.
- Storage suppositories should be protected from heat, preferably by storing in the refrigerator. Store in a cool place or refrigerator for external use only.
- **Testing/evaluation of suppositories finished suppositories are routinely inspected for:** Appearance. Content uniformity melting range test breaking test drug release test disintegration test dissolution testing liquefaction or softening time.

PRACTICE QUESTIONS
SHORT ANSWER TYPE QUESTIONS

1. Define the term 'suppository'.
2. Explain the term 'displacement value'.
3. Name the different types of suppositories which are available in the market.
4. Write the various types of lubricants used to lubricate the suppository mould.
5. Why cocoa butter is not used in the preparation of suppositories.
6. Mention different methods of preparation of suppositories.
7. What is the importance of calibration of the mould?
8. Write the advantages and disadvantages of suppositories.
9. Mention the qualities of an ideal suppository base.
10. Write in brief, the advantages and disadvantages of theobroma oil as suppository base?
11. What are the advantages and disadvantages of hydrogenated oil as suppository base?

LONG ANSWER TYPE QUESTIONS

1. What are 'suppositories'? Classify different suppository bases used in the preparation of suppositories. Describe briefly each base.
2. Define the term 'suppositories'. What are the advantages and disadvantages of suppositories?
3. What do you mean by 'suppositories'? Describe in brief the various types of suppositories.
4. Discuss in brief, the various methods of preparation of suppositories.
5. Write short notes on the following:
   a. Theobroma oil
   b. Displacement value
   c. Pessaries
   d. Fusion method of preparation of suppositories.

6. What is an advantage of the oleaginous bases with regards to membrane tissues?

7. Describe the procedure used for melting cocoa butter.

8. What release characteristics would one expect to be associated with hydrophobic drugs and oleaginous suppository bases?

9. What do PEG suppository bases do when inserted into the body?

10. List three advantages and disadvantages of PEG suppository bases.

11. Enumerate various factors to consider when selecting a suppository base?

12. What is the rationale for recommending that patients moisten PEG suppositories (e) prior to insertion?

13. What type of base is preferred when an emollient effect is desired?

14. What are the two methods used for compounding suppositories?

15. Why are density calculations and mold calibration so important when (f) compounding suppositories using the fusion method?

16. Define the term density displacement factor?

17. Perform the calculations for preparing 10 suppositories each containing 180 mg of phenobarbital as the sole active ingredient and using cocoa butter as your base.
(g) Your mold has been calibrated and the average weight per suppository is 2 g.

OBJECTIVE TYPE QUESTION

1. Suppositories are .... dosage form of drugs.

2. Suppositories are used to produce ...., ...
and .... action.

3. Cocoa butter is a mixture of .... of stearic, palmitic, oleic and other fatty acids.

4. In suppositories, the drug is released either due to .... of base or .... its contents in .... fluid.

5. Compression method is suitable for the preparation of suppositories containing .... and .... drugs.

6. Cocoa butter is not a suitable base for .... and .... suppositories.

Answers

1. Unit
2. Local, systemic mechanical
3. Glyceryl esters
4. Melting, dissolving, body cavity
5. Thermolabile, insoluble
6. Pessaries, nasal

Chapter 9

Dental Preparation

ORAL HYGIENE COSMETICS

Maintenance of health of the teeth and gums well is very important for having good general health. Health of teeth and gum of a person is an indication of his general health. So, it is necessary to take care of health of teeth and gums. Various preparations are used for cleansing and maintenance of good health of teeth, gum and oral cavity. The products, termed dentifrices are used to keep the teeth clean, shiny and to inhibit the formation of unpleasant odour in mouth and freshen the breath.

Oral hygiene cosmetics are:

1. Dentifrices
2. Toothpaste
3. Tooth powder
4. Mouthwash.

Dentifrices

Maintenance of teeth clean and in good health is essential and also important for everyone. This can be achieved by using various dental care preparations or dentifrices. Dentifrices are the preparations used for cleaning the surfaces of teeth and keep them shiny and to preserve the health of the teeth and gums (Fig. 9.1). These preparations may also expected to help inhibit the formation of unpleasant odours and freshen the breath. Regular use of dentifrices helps to prevent occurrence

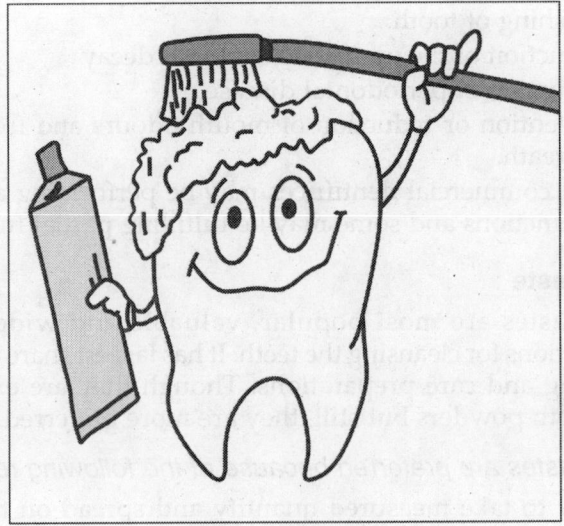

Fig. 9.1: Dentifrices

of tooth decay. A good dental health increases the possibility of a good general health.

Dentifrices can be either simple cleansing dentifrices or also be therapeutic dentifrices. Therapeutic dentifrices are basically cleansing preparations containing additionally, some drugs or chemicals which decreases the occurrence of dental caries or help in control of periodontal disease. These are achieved by the bactericidal, bacteriostatic, enzyme-inhibiting or acid-neutralizing qualities of the drugs or chemicals used. Therapeutic dentifrices containing stannous fluoride are widely used products.

Dentifrices are prepared in paste, powder and to a lesser extent in liquid and block forms.

Functions of Dentifrices

Though the primary function of a dentifrice is the cleaning of the accessible surfaces of the teeth, but it can have some other functions also. The expected functions of a dentifrice are as follows:

  i. Cleansing of tooth
 ii. Prevention of formation or removal of dental plaque
iii. Prevention of formation of calculus

iv. Polishing of tooth
v. Reduction of the occurrence of tooth decay
vi. Reduction of periodontal disease
vii. Prevention or reduction of mouth odours and freshening of breath.

Some commercial dentifrices may be performing all of the above functions and some may be fulfilling partial functions.

Toothpaste

Toothpastes are most popular, valuable and widely used preparations for cleansing the teeth. It has largest share of dental cleansing and care preparations. Though they are expensive than tooth powders but still, they are more preferred.

Toothpastes are preferred because of the following reasons:

1. Easy to take measured quantity and spread on the tooth brush.
2. No spillage or wastage.
3. Attractive consistency.
4. Proper distribution in mouth.

Formulae of Toothpaste

Ingredients	%w/w
Calcium carbonate	50–60
Sodium lauryl sulphate	0.5–1.5
Glycerine	20–26
Gum tragacanth	1–2
Water	17–20
Saccharine	0.1–0.3
Flavour	q.s
Preservative	q.s

Manufacturing Process

These preparations are preferably made in stainless steel mixer container. It can be done in a planetary mixer or similar mixer used for semisolid preparations. Small scale batch can be made in a glass container.

The gum is mixed with a suitable quantity of humectant, without any water for proper dispersion. Chloroform or alcohol can also be used for dispersion of binding agents. Other colloids may be dispersed in water. Preservative can be dissolved in glycerine or water. Methyl cellulose should be mixed with cold water, but ethyl cellulose should be dispersed in warm water. Other powder ingredients are sifted together and added gradually to mucilaginous mixture with continuous gentle stirring. Then aqueous media is mixed and stirred further to get the product. Favour and detergent should be added at the last.

In an alternative method the binder is premixed with solid abrasives and other powders and then poured in a suitable mixer (dough-type mixer) along with aqueous solution of the humectant, preservative, sweetening agent and mixing is done. After obtaining a homogeneous paste, flavour and detergent are added (Flowchart 9.1).

Tooth Powder

Tooth powders are, structurally, the oldest and simplest preparations and they are also the cheapest. Over the years their market share has been reduced by popularity and advantages of pastes, but still they have a considerable share of the market and population. The main problems encountered with tooth powders are floating of powders in air during manufacturing, formation of cake on storage, and uneven

Flowchart 9.1: Manufacturing process of toothpaste

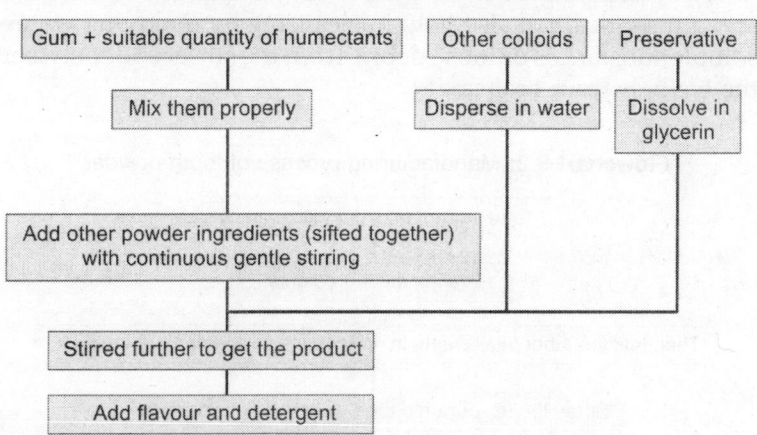

distribution in mouth. The oldest tooth powder is reported to be camphorated chalk. More or less every dental care manufacturer also markets tooth powders along with toothpaste products.

Formulae of Tooth Powder

Ingredients	%w/w
Calcium carbonate	80–85
Tricalcium phosphate	5–15
Sodium lauryl sulphate	1–5
Sodium perborate	1–5
Saccharine sodium	1–2
Flavour	q.s
Colour	q.s

Manufacturing Process

This is done by simple mixing. First ingredients of small quantity are premixed and then mixed with other ingredients in ribbon-type or agitator type of mixer. Flavour can be sprayed onto the bulk or can be premixed with part of some abrasive and polishing agent and then mixed with the bulk (Flowchart 9.2).

Mouthwash

Mouthwashes are basically deodorants and antiseptics. Mouthwashes, apart from their main function of deodorants and antiseptics, can also help in cleansing by removing water-soluble substances or loose debris from the surfaces or between the teeth or from oral cavity.

Flowchart 9.2: Manufacturing process of tooth powder

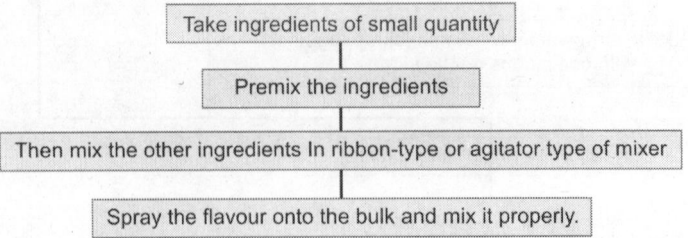

Mouthwashes are mainly alcoholic or hydroalcoholic solution as they are used in oral cavity, which need to be suitably diluted if required (Fig. 9.2)

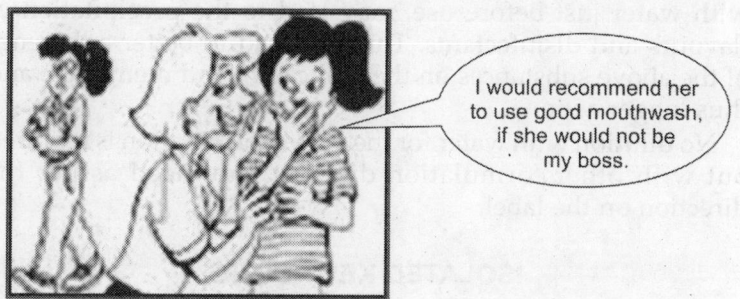

Fig. 9.2: Mouthwash is used to enhance oral hygiene

Mouthwash should have the following characters:

i. Good and quick antiseptic action at the dilution it is used
ii. Attractive flavour to impart a odour to the mouth
iii. Sweet taste
iv. Not much expensive
v. Non-irritant and non-toxic to mouth and mucous membrane.

I would recommend her to use good mouthwash, if she would not be my boss.

Formulae of Mouthwash

Ingredients	% w/w
Anethol	0.5–1
Methyl salicylate	05–1.5
Menthol	0.1–0.5
Propylene glycol	20–30
Glycerine	20–30
Tween 80	15–25
Saccharin sodium	1–3
Ethyl alcohol	22–30
Colour	q.s

Application of Mouthwash

The preparation is to be diluted with water in definite proportion, as suggested on the label, before use.

Dilution with water may have another advantage as dilution with water just before use, may lead to the precipitation of flavours and disinfectants. This will lead to better adherence of the above substances on the oral cavity and membrane and thus longer action.

No dilution with water for the above formulation is required but with other formulation dilution may need as per the direction on the label.

ISOLATED KEY POINTS

- Cosmetics arise from a greek word kosmeticos which means adorn.
- Dentifrices are used to keep the teeth clean, shiny and to inhibit the formation of unpleasant odour in mouth and freshen the breath.
- Oral hygiene cosmetics are:
    - i. Dentifrices
    - ii. Toothpaste
    - iii. Tooth powder
    - iv. Mouthwash
- Toothpastes are most popular, valuable and widely used preparations for cleansing the teeth.
- Tooth powders are, structurally, the oldest and simplest preparations and they are also the cheapest.
- Mouthwashes are basically deodorants and antiseptics. Mouthwashes, apart from their main function of deodorants and antiseptics, can also help in cleansing by removing water-soluble substances or loose debris from the surfaces or between the teeth or from oral cavity.
- Mouthwashes are mainly alcoholic or hydroalcoholic solution as they are used in oral cavity, which need to be suitably diluted if required.

LONG ANSWER TYPE QUESTIONS

1. What do you understand by the term cosmetics? Elaborate in detail about the applications of cosmetics in the healthcare systems.

2. What are dentifrices? Write in detail about the role of dentifrices.

3. What are hair dressings? Give suitable example of hair dressings.

4. What are hair removers? Explain various methods used for removing hair with suitable examples.

SHORT ANSWER TYPE QUESTIONS

1. Substances which are intended to be applied to the human body for cleansing, beautifying, promoting attractiveness, or altering the appearance without affecting the body's structure or functions are called ....

2. Hair .... are used after shampooing the hair, to render the hair more lustrous, easy to comb, and free from static electricity when dry.

3. Which of the following is not the function of hair:
   a. Hair on the head protect the scalp from ultraviolet light, cushion round the head and insulate the skull
   b. Eyebrows protect the eye from small foreign particles and insects
   c. Body hair helps in biochemical synthesis of vitamins
   d. The hairs, guarding the entrances to nostrils and external ear canals filter the air and help prevent the entry of foreign particles

4. Which of the following is not an oral hygiene cosmetic:
   a. Dentifrices
   b. Toothpaste
   c. Gargle
   d. Mouthwash

Answers

1. Cosmetics
2. Conditioners
3. c
4. c

Chapter 10

Cosmetic Preparation

Cosmetics are substances used to enhance the appearance or odour of the human body. They are generally mixtures of chemical compounds, some being derived from natural sources, many being synthetic.

In the US, the Food and Drug Administration (FDA) which regulates cosmetics, defines cosmetics as "intended to be applied to the human body for cleansing, beautifying, promoting attractiveness, or altering the appearance without affecting the body's structure or functions." This broad definition includes, as well, any material intended for use as a component of a cosmetic product.

The cosmetics are mainly external or topical preparations and are meant to be applied to external parts of the body. In other words they may be applied to skin, hair and nails for the purposes of covering, colouring, softening, cleansing, nourishing, waving, setting, mollification, preservation, removal and protection.

Types of Skin

There are five basic skin types, including:

Normal Skin

This type of skin has a fine, even and smooth surface due to having an ideal balance between oil and moisture contents and is therefore, neither greasy nor dry. People who have normal skin have small, barely-visible pores. Thus, their skin appears clear and does not develop spots and blemishes. This type of skin needs minimal and gentle treatment.

Dry Skin

Dry skin has a parched appearance and tends to flake easily. It is prone to wrinkles and lines due to the inability to retain moisture, as well as, the inadequate production of sebum by sebaceous glands. Dry skin often has problems in cold weather as it dries up even further. Constant protection in the form of a moisturizer by day and a moisture-rich cream by night is essential.

Oily Skin

As its name implies, this type of skin's surface is slightly to moderately greasy, which is caused by the over secretion of sebum. The excess oil on the surface of the skin draws dirt and dust from the environment to stick to it. Oily skin is usually prone to black heads, white heads, spots and pimples. It needs to be cleansed thoroughly everyday.

Combination Skin

This is the most common type of skin. As the name suggests, it is a combination of both oily and dry skin where certain areas of the face are oily and the rest dry. The oily parts are usually found on a central panel, called T—Zone, consisting of the forehead, nose and chin. The dry areas consist of the cheeks and the areas around the eyes and mouth. In such cases, each part of the face should be treated accordingly where the dry areas are treated as for dry skin and the central panel is treated as for oily skin. There are also skin care products made especially for those who have combination skin.

Sensitive Skin

Sensitive skin has a very fine texture and is excessively sensitive to changes in the climate. This skin type is easily irritated, bruised and/or scarred from bleaching, waxing, threading, perfumes, temperature extremes, soap, shaving creams, etc. People who belong to this skin type should avoid products with dyes, perfumes, or unnecessary chemical ingredients that may aggravate the skin.

Classification of Skin Cosmetics

1. Skin cosmetics
2. Hair cosmetics

3. Nails cosmetics

4. Oral hygiene cosmetics

All cosmetics are formulated as solids, semisolids or liquids. Their formula design is very similar to drug dosage forms.

Skin cosmetics: Skin cosmetics include:

1. Powder

2. Lipstick

3. Cold cream

4. Shaving preparation

5. Antiperspirant and deodorant

POWDERS

Face Powder

Face powder is basically a cosmetic product which has as its prime function the ability to complement skin colour by imparting a velvet finish to it (Fig. 10.1).

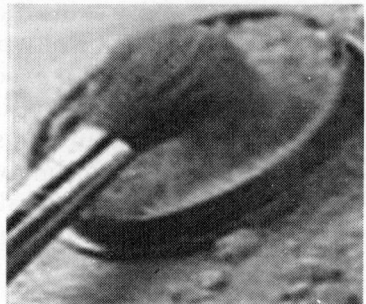

Fig. 10.1: Face powder

Desired Characteristics or Attributes of Face Powder

A good face powder should have following attributes:

1. It should produce a smooth finish to the facial skin

2. Mask visible imperfections of the face

3. Shine due to moisture or grease from perspiration or secretion of sebaceous and sweat glands or from preparations used on the skin.

4. The powder must produce a lasting effect, so that frequent application is unnecessary.

5. The preparation should make the face pleasant to look and touch. The degree of opacity can vary from opaque, in case of clown make-up, to almost transparent.
6. It must adhered to the skin and be reasonably resistant to the mixed secretion of the skin.

Example Formulae of Face Powders

Ingredients	% w/w
Talc	50–70
Kaolin	15–25
Calcium carbonate (light)	5–7
Zinc oxide	5–9
Zinc stearate	2–8
Magnesium carbonates	0.5–1.5
Colour	0.1–0.9
Perfume	0.1–0.9

Manufacturing process

The preparation of powders is simple as it is simply a matter of dry mixing of finely powdered materials. Add the perfume with part of the absorbent materials like calcium carbonate or with magnesium carbonate and keep it aside for some time. Mix the colour with part of the talc properly and add the other powders and then the perfume mixture. Mix and sieve the powder mixture using a silk mesh or an old washed nylon cloth (Flowchart 10.1).

Flowchart 10.1: Manufacturing process of face powder

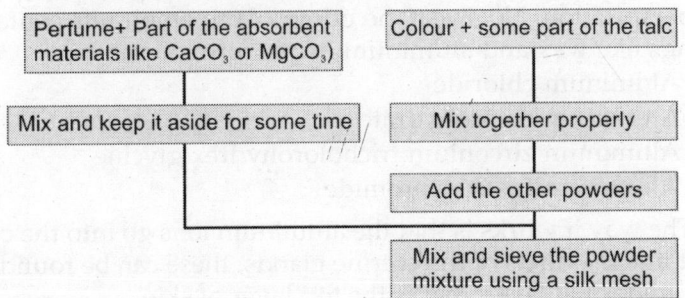

Body Powder

Amongst the various cosmetics, body powder is one of the widely consumed cosmetic preparations. Body powders are also known as **talcum powders or dusting powders**.

Purpose of using body powder: The main use of body powders or talcum powders is to absorb moisture or perspiration specifically after bathing particularly in warmer countries. These also provide good slip, a cooling effect and efficient lubrication, and prevent irritation of skin due to chafing. The very fine particle size of these covers a large surface area per unit weight and can cover a large body area which results in strong light dispersion and therefore, visual covering of the skin underneath.

The surface covered by the powders is much more than the surface uncovered which leads to a cooling effect, if the ingredients of the powder have good heat conductivity. These fine powder particles with light weight adhere to the skin by the stickiness of the fat film.

Antiperspirant and Deodorant (Figs 10.2 and 10.3)

Most people think that antiperspirants and deodorants are the same thing, but they are not.

The fundamental differences lie in the way these products work, and potentially affect health. Essentially, they each use different chemical processes for minimizing body odour. Certain ingredients in either product may be unhealthy, but deodorant is frequently cited as a better alternative than many antiperspirants.

Antiperspirants contain fragrance, but they also contain chemical compounds that block the pores to stop the discharge of perspiration. No sweat, no odour. Antiperspirants contains things like wax and aluminum in one form or another.

a. Aluminum chloride
b. Aluminum chlorohydrate
c. Aluminum zirconium tricholorohydrex glycine
d. Aluminum hydroxybromide

The way it works is that the aluminum ions go into the cells that line the ducts of the eccrine glands, these can be found on the epidermal layer, that is the top layer of skin.

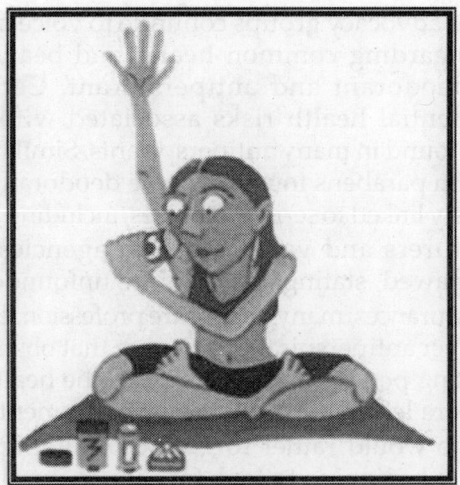

Fig. 10.2: Women using antiperspirant stick

Deodorant allows the release of perspiration, but prevents odour by combating it with antiseptic agents, which kill odour-causing bacteria.

Many consumers do not realize how deodorant works, assuming it is simply a fragrance that covers up body odour. Some choose antiperspirant, because rather than cover the odour, they prefer to eliminate it.

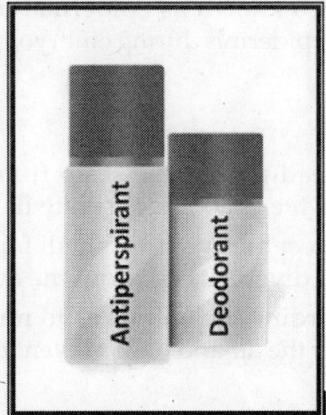

Fig. 10.3: Antiperspirant and deodorant spray

Consumer advocacy groups continue to voice concerns over questions regarding common health and beauty products, including deodorant and antiperspirant. Certain studies indicate potential health risks associated with aluminium compounds found in many antiperspirants. Similar studies find like risks with parabens found in some deodorants. Both have been tenuously linked to serious illnesses, including breast cancer.

Manufacturers and various health agencies claim such studies are flawed, stating concerns are unfounded.

Despite assurances, many healthcare professionals recommend deodorant over antiperspirant, believing that obstructing pores and preventing perspiration may not be the healthiest choice. Consumers are left to make their own judgements.

Those who would rather forgo a typical antiperspirant or deodorant are beginning to look for more natural alternatives. There are several brands of natural deodorant that are currently available. However, these products do not always contain purely organic ingredients, so check labels carefully before purchasing. For the true maverick, a homespun deodorant consists of equal parts cornstarch and baking soda, applied with a damp washcloth.

Hair Cosmetics

To study and design hair preparations it is very much essential to have knowledge of hair. Hair is one of the vital parts of the body. They are also known as epidermal derivatives as they originate from the epidermis during embryological development (Fig. 10.4).

Functions of Hair

1. Hair on the head protect the scalp from ultraviolet light, cushion round the head and insulate the skull.

2. Eyebrows protect the eye from small foreign particles and insects. Also it diverts sweat from the eyes.

3. The hairs, guarding the entrances to nostrils and external ear canals filter the air and help prevent the entry of foreign Particles.

4. Body hair helps in evaporation of perspiration and draining of external water from the body.

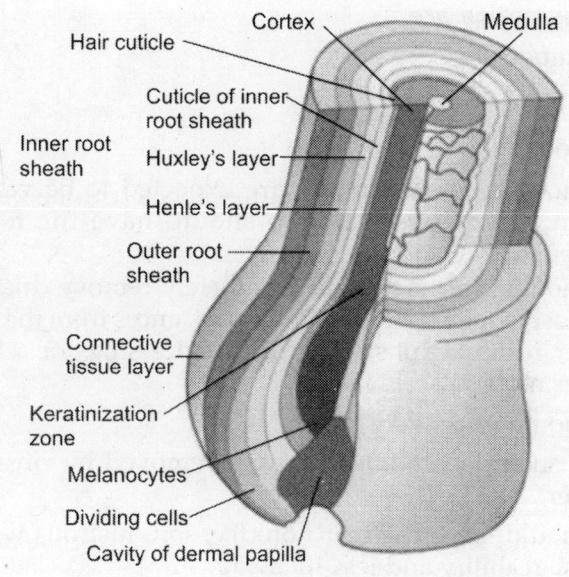

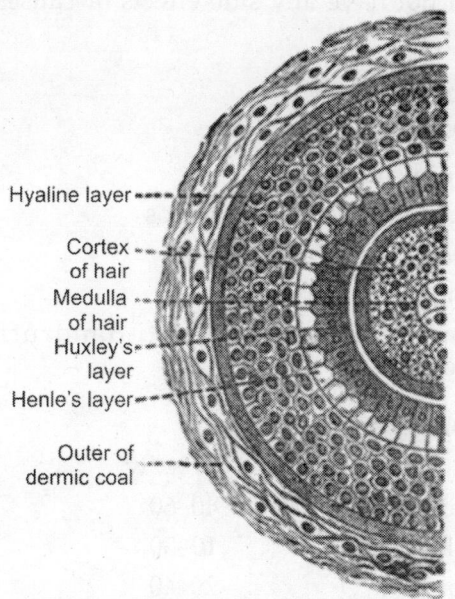

Fig. 10.4: Schematic structure of hair

Hair Cosmetics are

1. Shampoo
2. Conditioner

Shampoo

The functions of a shampoo are expected to be various. A good an acceptable shampoo should have the following characteristics:

i. It should effectively and completely remove dust or soil, excessive sebum or other fatty substances from the hair and other residual substances of hair dressings or settings or other materials.

ii. It should effectively wash the hair.

iii. The shampoo should be easily removed by rinsing with water.

iv. It should leave the hair non-dry, soft, lustrous with good manageability and less fly away.

v. It should impart a pleasant fragrance to the hair.

vi. It should not have any side effects or causes irritation to skin or eye.

Types of Shampoo

1. Powder shampoos
2. Clear liquid shampoos
3. Liquid cream or lotion shampoos
4. Solid cream/gel shampoos
5. Oil shampoos
6. Miscellaneous including anti-dandruff medicated shampoos.

Formulae of Powder Shampoos

Ingredients	% w/w
Sodium bicarbonate	40–60
Disodium phosphate	10–30
Soap powder	20–40
Perfume	q.s

Manufacturing Process

They are prepared by simple mixing process. In powder shampoos the ingredients are simply mixed and the perfume is added last (Flowchart 10.2).

Flowchart 10.2: Manufacturing process of powder shampoos

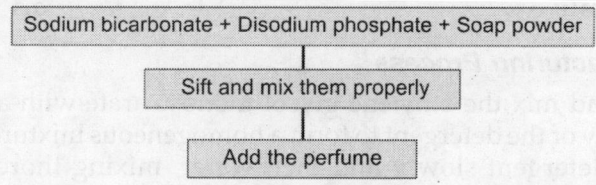

Formulae of Clear Liquid Shampoos

Ingredients	% w/w
Triethanolamine lauryl sulphate	40–50
Coconut monoethanolamide	1–3
Water	50–56
Perfume	q.s
Colour	q.s
Preservative	q.s

Manufacturing Process

In case of clear liquid shampoos the detergents are first dissolved in half of the water with little heat if necessary. Other ingredients are added to other part of the water and then mixed with the first part. The perfume is added at last (Flowchart 10.3).

Flowchart 10.3: Manufacturing process of clear liquid shampoos

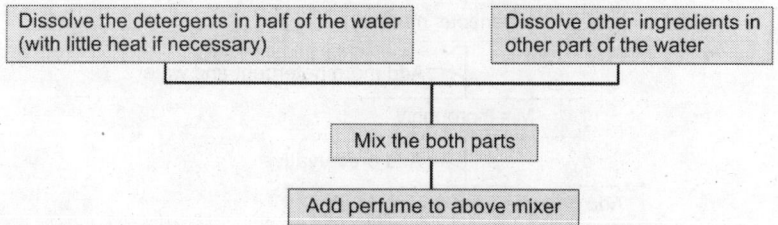

Formulae of Liquid cream or lotion shampoos

Ingredients	% w/w
Monoethanolamine lauryl sulphate (25% active)	30–50
Ethylene glycol monostearate	3–7
Water	50–60
Perfume	q.s
Preservative	q.s

Manufacturing Process

Heat and mix the ethylene glycol monostearate with a small quantity of the detergent to form a homogeneous mixture. Add more detergent slowly and then water, mixing thoroughly before addition of next. Perfume is added last after cooling to 35°C (Flowchart 10.4).

Formulae of Solid cream/Gel Shampoos

Ingredients	g/batch
Sodium lauryl sulphate	15–25
Coconut monsethanolamide	0.5–1.5
Propylene glycol monostearate	1–3
Stearic acid	3–7
Sodium hydroxide	0.5–1
Water	65–75
Perfume	q.s

Flowchart 10.4: Manufacturing process of lotion shampoos

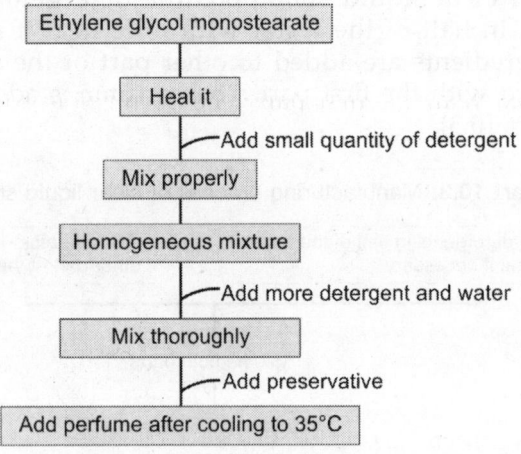

Manufacturing Process

Mix water, oleic acid and sodium lauryl sulphate paste and heat to 60°C. Slowly add triethanolamine with continuous stirring. Add perfume after cooling to 35°C (Flowchart 10.5)

Flowchart 10.5: Manufacturing process of gel shampoos

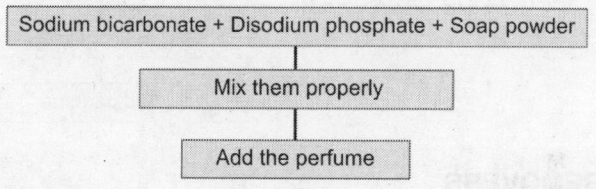

Conditioner

Conditioners are used after shampooing the hair, to render the hair more lustrous, easy to comb, and free from static electricity when dry. They are also used to improve damaged hair. Hair may be damaged by excessive use of bleaches and permanent waves. Conditioners are usually based on cationic detergents and fatty materials like lanolin or mineral oil.

Formulae of Conditioner

Ingredients	% w/w
Stearyl alcohol	0.25–.75
Glyceryl monostearate	2–6
Sodium chloride	0.1–0.3
Benzalkonium chloride	1–2
Water	95–99
Colour	q.s
Perfume	q.s

Manufacturing Process

Dissolve the sodium chloride in a small quality of water with heating at 75°C. Add colour to the sodium chloride solution. Take glyceryl monostearate and stearic acid together and mix with heating at about 60°C and then add to the aqueous solution. Stir and cool and add perfume and preservative (Flowchart 10.6).

Flowchart 10.6: Manufacturing process of conditioner

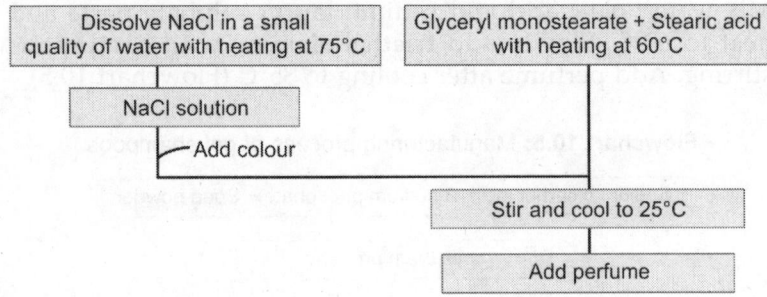

HAIR REMOVERS

Many people have unwanted hair. It is common on the upper lip, chin, cheeks, back, legs, fingers, feet, and toes. It can have many causes, including genetics, certain medications, such as steroids, higher levels of certain hormones, and polycystic ovarian syndrome.

Hair removers, or depilatories, are products designed to chemically or physically remove undesirable hair from areas on the body.

Hair removal, also known as epilation or depilation, is the deliberate removal of body hair.

Hair can become more visible during and after puberty and men tend to have thicker, more visible body hair than women. Both men and women have visible hair on the head, eyebrows, eyelashes, armpits, pubic region, arms, and legs; men and some women also have thicker hair on their face, abdomen, back and chest. Hair does not generally grow on the lips, the underside of the hands or feet or on certain areas of the genitalia.

Forms of hair removal are practised for various and mostly cultural, sexual, medical or religious reasons. Forms of hair removal have been practiced in almost all human cultures since, at least the neolithic era. The methods used to remove hair have varied in different times and regions, but shaving is the most common method. There are several ways to remove unwanted hair

Shaving

Shaving is best for leg, arm, and facial hair. It can, though, cause ingrown hairs, especially in the pubic region.

Plucking

Plucking or tweezing can be painful, but it may be a good option when only few hairs are to be removed. Used to pluck hairs from eyebrows or pulling out a few stray hairs that appear on the face.

Depilatory Creams

Hair removal creams, also known as depilatory creams, are available without a prescription.

They are not all the same, so be sure to read the label. For instance, a hair removal cream made for pubic hairs should not be used to remove hair on the face.

The chemicals in these products dissolve the hair shaft. Using a cream improperly for instance, leaving it on too long can burn the skin.

Hot Waxing

Hot waxing can be messy and painful and may leave some hairs behind because they can break off. If the wax is too hot, it may cause a burn. Generally women use this hair removal method in the bikini area and to remove hair on the upper lip.

Threading

Threading is a traditional Indian method of hair removal that some salons offer. The professionals who do threading use strings they twist in a pattern and use to pull unwanted hair out.

Laser Hair Removal

This is one of the longest lasting methods, but it generally requires four or more treatments 4–6 weeks apart. It can only be effective on dark hair.

The laser beam is used to destroy the hair bulb, the treatment is expensive and sometimes painful, but it can be used on many parts of the body where unwanted hair appears. Done by professional doctor or technician who is highly trained.

Electrolysis

Electrolysis is done by a professional who places a tiny needle with an electric current in the hair follicle. There are two primary hair removal methods with electrolysis: galvanic and thermolytic.

i. Galvanic hair removal chemically destroys the hair follicle.

ii. Thermolytic removal uses heat to destroy the follicle.

Done by professional doctor or technician who is highly trained. It can be done on any part of the body.

Medications and Unwanted Hair

If none of these hair removal methods help, one should take doctor's advice. There are drugs that inhibit hair growth.

Spironolactone is a pill that may slow or reduce hair growth in areas that you do not want hair. It will not get rid of the hair on scalp. There is a prescription cream called Vaniqa that's approved by the FDA for slowing facial hair growth in women. This cream slows growth, but it will not remove the hair. It is to be applied to the area twice a day.

Disadvantages

There are several disadvantages of hair removal methods.

i. Hair removal can cause skin inflammation, minor burns, lesions, scarring, ingrown hairs, bumps, and infected hair follicles.

ii. Some removal methods are not permanent, can cause medical problems and permanent damage, or have very high costs.

ISOLATED KEY POINTS

- Cosmetics arise from a greek word *kosmeticos* which means adorn. If any material used for beautification or improvement of appearance is known as cosmetics. In other words they may be applied to skin, hair and nails for the purpose of covering colouring, softening, cleansing, nourishing, setting and protection.

- Classification of cosmetics skin hair nail hygienic powder compact creams lotion colourants hair remover, hair conditioner shampoos hair dyes, lotion eyelash (mascaras) eyebrow pencils eyelid inside (kohls) face powder compact powder body powder prickly heat powder cold cream vanishing cream all purpose cream cleansing cream foundation cream emollient cream astringent lotion lip sticks rouges nail lacquers lacquer removers nail polish cuticle removers DENTAL powders paste dentifrices lotion mouth wash BATH soap bath.

- Skin introduction skin is the heaviest single organ of the body combine with the mucosal lining of the respiratory, digestive and urogenital tract. A square centimeter of skin covers 10 hair follicles, 12 nerves, 15 sebaceous gland, 100 sweat gland. PH of the skin varies from 4–5.6.

- Function of the skin: Protection from external stimuli like chemicals, light, heat and cold, radiation. It regulates the body temperature controlling blood pressure. It acts as a barrier for invasions of various microorganisms. It has bactericidal fungicidal activities due to presence of sebum secretion. It has an important role in the synthesis of vitamin D_3—Calcitriol.

- The human skin consists of mainly three types, there are epidermis, dermis and subcutaneous.

- Epidermis: It is multilayer. It varies in thickness, depends on cell size and area, such as soles, palm – 0.8 mm eyelid –0.06 mm. The epidermis comprise 5 distinct layers— Stratum corneum (horny layer), Stratum lucidum, Stratum granulosum (granular layer) Stratum spinosum (prickly cell layer), Stratum germinativum (basal layer).

  - **Stratum corneum:** It consist of epidermal cells lipophilic nature the membrane provides about 10–15 layers of flattened keratinized dead cells It is 10 um when it is dry. But it can take up moisture up to 15–20%. When occlusive dressing/cream applied over the skin prevent the evaporation of water it plays a role in controlling the percutaneous absorption of chemical substance.

  - **Stratum lucidum:** It is thin translucent layer stratum granulosum: It is consist of keratin protein stratum spinosum: it consist of flattened polygonal cells stratum germinativum: it consist of melanocytes.

- Dermis/corium it consist of dense network of structural protein fibres—collagen. Mucopolysaccharide–ground substance It is about 0.2–0.3 mm thickness It contains blood vessels, lymphatic vessels, nerve ending.

- Subcutaneous it consist of fat rich areolar tissue. It is otherwise called superficial fascia. It is quite elastic. Large arteries and vein are present.
- **Skin appendages sebaceous gland hair follicle/pile pilosebaceous unit sweat gland:** Eccrine gland/salty sweat gland–present overall body surface apocrine gland–axillae, anogenital region, around nipple. Sebaceous gland–secretes sebum (waxes, sterols, f. acid).
- Skin powders are widely used for face and body care not only for woman but also for men. Powders are differ from liquid skin care ppn, e.g. body powder/talcum powder/ dusting powder very fine powder can cover large surface area of the body.
- Ideal character of powder should be good covering power and hide skin blemishes should adhere to the skin and not blow of easily should not completely dissipated in a few minutes to avoid repowdering. The finish given to the skin must be preferably peach like character. Shine on around the nose must be completely eliminated. Must be absorbent. Must be slip enable the powder to spread on the skin by the puff.
- Face powder face powder is a basically a cosmetic product which imparts velvet like finish to it. A good face powder should produce smooth finish to facial skin masking visible imperfection of the face and shine due to moisture or grease or oily secretion. The preparation should make the face pleasant look and touch. It must adhere to the skin and mixed secretion of skin.
- **Body powder:** It is called talcum powder/dusting powder. They are used as multiple purpose. It is use to absorb moisture or perspiration specific after bath. It is also act as cooling effect and prevent irritation of skin due to chafing. It contains covering material, adhesive, absorbancy material, slip antiseptic and perfumes. It consist of small portion of metallic stearate and talc, ppt chalk. A. Septic material used to proliferation of microbes.

LONG ANSWER TYPE QUESTIONS

1. What do you understand by the term cosmetics? Elaborate in detail about the applications of cosmetics in the healthcare systems.

2. Define the face powders. Write in detail about the manufacturing process evolved in the face powder manufacturing.

3. How face powder can enhance the appearance of the skin? Write comments.

4. Differentiate between the face powder and body Powder.

5. What do you mean by the word "Lip sticks"? How you will prepare it? Write in detail about the precautions taken while manufacturing lip sticks?

6. Write the ideal formula to prepare the lip sticks.

7. What do you mean by the term "cold creams"? Discuss its role in cosmetology.

8. Define cold creams. Discuss its manufacturing process with the with the help of suitable flow charts.

9. Cold cream is o/w or w/o type emulsion. Explain with the formula.

10. How vanishing creams are different from cold creams?

11. What do you mean by all purpose creams? Explain the manufacturing process and applications of all purpose creams.

12. Define shaving cream. Discuss in detail about the role of key ingredients of the shaving cream.

13. How the deodorants are different from the antiperspirants? Explain by using suitable example.

14. How deodorants are useful in the management of the bad odour? Explain their mechanism.

15. Write the advantage and disadvantage of deodorants usage.

16. Define shampoo. Explain its manufacturing process.

17. Discuss in brief:
    a. Clear liquid shampoo
    b. Gel shampoos
    c. Oil shampoos
    d. Antiseptic/antidandruff shampoo

18. What do you mean by the word "conditioners"? How it is different from shampoo, explain with the formula?

19. What are hair dressings? Give suitable example of hair dressings.

20. What are hair removers? Explain various methods used for removing hair with suitable examples.

SHORT ANSWER TYPE QUESTIONS

1. Substances which are intended to be applied to the human body for cleansing, beautifying, promoting attractiveness, or altering the appearance without affecting the body's structure or functions are called ....

2. There are various layers of cells within the epidermis, the outermost layer of skin is called ....

3. Vanishing cream are .... type emulsion, as name indicates these creams get.................... after applied and rubbed onto the skin.

4. .... contain fragrance, but they also block the pores to stop the discharge of perspiration while .... allows the release of perspiration, but prevents odour by combating it with antiseptic agents, which kill odour-causing bacteria.

5. Hair .... are used after shampooing the hair, to render the hair more lustrous, easy to comb, and free from static electricity when dry.

6. Which of the following is false in context to function of skin:
   a. Protects the body against physical injury and microbes
   b. Homeostatis
   c. Provides protection from UV light.
   d. Vitamin E synthesis and biotransformation of some chemicals

7. Cold cream is:
   a. W/o emulsion
   b. W/o/w emulsion
   c. Provides protection from UV light
   d. Forms a dry layer on skin

8. To remove the make up and foundation bases cream used is:
   a. Vanishing cream
   b. Cleansing cream
   c. Moisturizer
   d. Cold cream

9. Which of the following is not the function of hair:
   a. Hair on the head protect the scalp from ultraviolet light, cushion round the head and insulate the skull
   b. Eyebrows protect the eye from small foreign particles and insects
   c. Body hair helps in biochemical synthesis of vitamins
   d. The hairs, guarding the entrances to nostrils and external ear canals filter the air and help prevent the entry of foreign particles

10. Which of the following is not an oral hygiene cosmetic:
    a. Dentifrices
    b. Toothpaste
    c. Gargle
    d. Mouthwash

Answers

1. Cosmetics
2. Stratum corneum (or horny layer)
3. O/w, disappeared
4. Antiperspirants, deodorant
5. Conditioners
6. d
7. a
8. b
9. c
10. c

Chapter 11

Parenteral Dosage form and Sterility Testing

DEFINITION

Parenteral (derived from Greek word, *para enteron,* beside the intestine) dosage forms of drugs are injected directly into body tissue through one or more layer of skin and mucous.

Advantages

- **Quick onset of action:** 15–30 seconds for IV, 3–5 minutes for IM and subcutaneous (subcut)
- 100% bioavailability for IV injection
- Suitable for drugs not absorbed by the gut or those that are too irritant (anti-cancer)
- One injection can be formulated to last days or even months, e.g. Depo-Provera, a birth control shot that works for three months
- IV can deliver continuous medication, e.g. morphine for patients in continuous pain, or saline drip and glucose for people needing fluids and nutrients
- Useful for unconscious and vomiting patient
- Suitable for drugs, which are inactivated by GIT fluid or enzymes.

Disadvantages

- Onset of action is quick, hence more risk of addiction when it comes to injecting drugs of abuse
- Patients are not typically able to self-administer, Need trained person

- Belonephobia, the fear of needles and injection
- If needles are shared, there is risk of HIV and other infectious diseases
- It is the most dangerous route of administration because it bypasses most of the body's natural defenses, exposing the user to health problems such as hepatitis, abscesses, infections, and undissolved particles or additives/contaminants
- If not done properly, potentially fatal air boluses (bubbles) can occur
- Need for strict asepsis.

Classifications

Parenteral dosage forms can be categorized in to six categories:
   i. Solutions ready for injection.
  ii. Dry, soluble products ready to be combined with a solvent just prior to use.
 iii. Suspensions ready for injection.
  iv. Dry insoluble products ready to be combined with a vehicle just prior to use.
   v. Emulsions.
  vi. Liquid concentrates ready for dilution prior to administration.

Routes of Administration (Table 11.1)

Types of Injections (Fig. 11.1)

Intradermal (in or into the skin): An intradermal injection is given into the skin. It is used for skin testing some allergens, and also for mantoux test for tuberculosis.

Subcutaneous: Under the skin. "Subcutaneous" implies just under the skin. With a subcutaneous injection, a needle is inserted just under the skin. A drug (e.g. insulin) can then be delivered into the subcutaneous tissues. After the injection, the drug moves into small blood vessels and the bloodstream. The subcutaneous route is used with many protein and polypeptide drugs, such as insulin which, if given by mouth, would be broken down and digested in the intestinal tract. The amount of medication is around 1 ml, given by holding the needle at 45° angle while piercing the skin, skin is pinched tight, insert needle so that hub of needle shaft touches the skin, aspirate to

Table 11.1: Various routes of administering parenteral drugs

Organs	*Injection type*
Skin	Intradermal
	Subcutaneous
Organs	Intracavernous
	Intravitreal
	Transscleral
Central nervous system	Intracerebral
	Intrathecal/intraspinal
	Epidural
	Intracisternal
Circulatory/musculoskeletal	Intravenous
	Intracardiac
	Intramuscular
	Intraosseous
	Intra-articular
	Intraperitoneal
	Intra-arterial

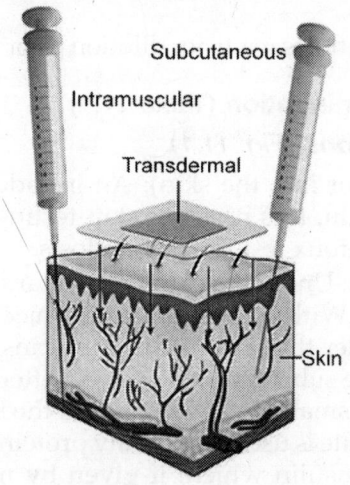

Fig. 11.1: Types of injections

check the location of needle. If blood is aspirated, withdraw the needle and try at other site, if not gently push the medication into subcutaneous tissue, withdraw needle and gently massage the area to help in absorption, never massage insulin or other drug which stains the skin.

Intracavernous: An intracavernous (or intracavernosal) injection is an injection into the base of the penis. This injection site is often used to administer medications to check for or treat erectile dysfunction in adult men.

Intravitreal: Intravitreal (Intravitreal is a route of administration of a drug, or other substance, in which the substance is delivered via an eye. "Intravitreal" literally means "inside an eye") (Fig. 11.2).

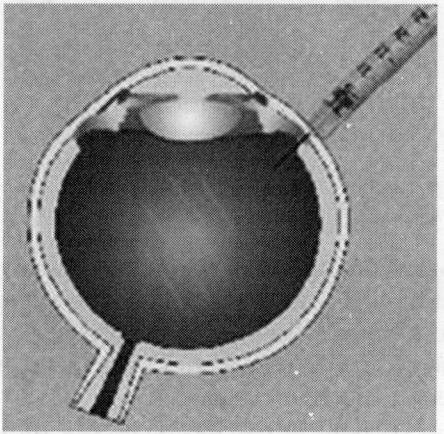

Fig. 11.2: Intravitreal injection

Transscleral (trans- + sclera + -al) Injected in to Sclera. (Sclera: The white of the eye. It is the tough outer coat of the eye that covers the eyeball except for the cornea.)

Intracerebral (L, intra + cerebrum, brain, pertaining to the area or substance within the cerebrum)—Injected in Cerebrum.

Intrathecal (**Intrathecal** (Latin intra- "inside", Greek theka "capsule", "hull") is an adjective that refers to something introduced into or occurring in the space under the arachnoid membrane of the spinal cord.) injection of a substance through the theca of the spinal cord into the subarachnoid space.

Epidural-injection of an anesthetic substance into the epidural space of the spinal cord in order to produce epidural anesthesia (Fig. 11.3).

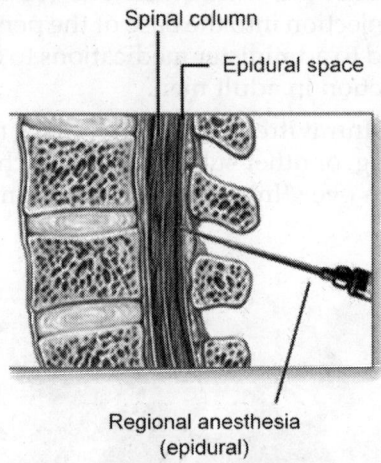

Spinal column

Epidural space

Regional anesthesia
(epidural)

Fig. 11.3: Epidural injection

Intraosseous infusion (into the bone marrow) is, in effect, an indirect intravenous access because the bone marrow drains directly into the venous system. This route is occasionally used for drugs and fluids in emergency medicine and pediatrics when intravenous access is difficult.

Intracisternal: It is given between the first and second cervical vertebrae—used to withdraw cerebrospinal fluid for diagnostic purposes.

Intravenous: Intravenous therapy or IV therapy is the giving of substances directly into a vein. The word intravenous simply means "within a vein".

Intracardiac: Intracardiac (into the heart), injection given into the heart, e.g. adrenaline during cardiopulmonary resuscitation, nowadays not commonly performed.

Intramuscular: Intramuscular injection into a muscle, e.g. many vaccines, antibiotics, and long-term psychoactive agents.

Intra-articular, (Origin: intra + L. Articulus, joint), drug injected with in joints (Fig. 11.4).

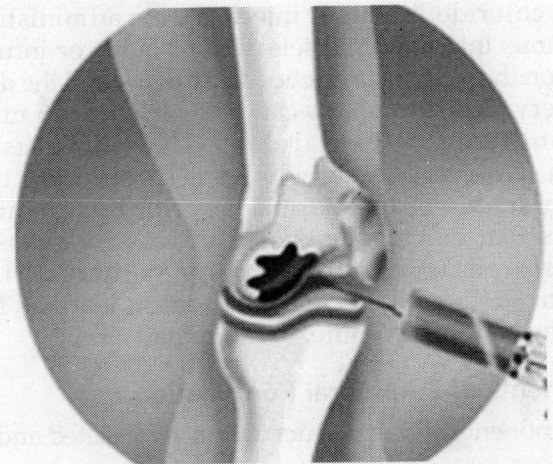

Fig. 11.4: Intra-articular injection

Intraperitoneal, (infusion or injection into the peritoneum): Intraperitoneal injection or IP injection is the injection of a substance into the peritoneum (body cavity). IP injection is more often applied to animals than humans, e.g. peritoneal dialysis.

Intra-arterial (arterial-arteries): Injected into arteries, e.g. vasodilator drugs in the treatment of vasospasm and thrombolytic drugs for treatment of embolism.

The most common routes of parenteral administration are intravenous (IV), subcutaneous (SC), and intramuscular (IM).

Classification on injections on the basis of injection volumes

Pharmacopoeias classify injectables into two on the basis of injection volumes

   i. Small-volume parenterals (SVPs)
  ii. Large-volume parenterals (LVPs).

Small-volume parenterals (SVPs): The US. Pharmacopoeia (USP) defines SVPs as containing less than 100 ml.

Large-volume parenterals (LVPs): The US. Pharmacopoeia (USP) defines LVPs as containing more than 100 ml.

SVPs given rapidly in a small volume are known as a bolus. SVPs may also be added to LVPs, such as 5% dextrose and 0.9%

sodium chloride infusion/injection, for administration by intravenous infusion. The selection of bolus or infusion will depend on the pharmacokinetics of the drug, and the distinction is not very clear. Infusions can be as brief as 15 minutes or may continue for several days. Usually infusions are formulated as a concentrate, which will subsequently be diluted by the practitioner or pharmacist prior to administration. Intramuscular or subcutaneous injections are almost always administered as a bolus. Usually volume of injection administered through subcutaneous route is less than 1 to 1.5 ml and for intramuscular route no more than 2 ml.

Components of Parenteral Formulation

The components of the product to be accumulated and selected include:

   i. Vehicles
   ii. Solute
   iii. Container
   iv. Closure

Vehicles

Majority of the injections are diluted so vehicle makes highest portion of the injection. Vehicles are categories in to following headings:

   i. Aqueous vehicles
   ii. Water-miscible vehicles
   iii. Nonaqueous vehicles.

   Aqueous vehicles: The vehicle of greatest importance is water, i.e. water for Injection (WFI). Usually aqueous vehicles are isotonic vehicles to which a drug may be added at the time of administration. For example, sodium chloride injection, Ringer's injection, dextrose injection, dextrose and sodium chloride injection, and lactated Ringer's injection.

Water for Injection

The USP monograph states: "Water for injection (WFI) is water purified by distillation or reverse osmosis."

WFI is produced by either distillation or 2 stage RO. It is usually stored and distributed hot (at 80°C) in order to meet microbial quality requirements and should not be used after 24 hours of storage.

Nonaqueous vehicles: The most important group of nonaqueous vehicles are the fixed oils. The fixed oils used in parenteral must be of vegetable origin because of following characteristics:

i. They will be metabolized
ii. Remain liquid at room temperature
iii. Will not become rancid readily.

The USP also specifies limits for the degree of unsaturation. and free fatty acid content. Examples of fixed oils are corn oil, cottonseed oil, peanut oil, and sesame oil. Fixed oils are used particularly as vehicles for certain hormone preparations and poorly soluble drugs for intramuscular administration can be formulated in a nonaqueous vehicle; this can have the additional benefit of providing a slow release of the active moiety. The label must state the name of the vehicle so that the user may beware in case of known sensitivity or other reactions to it.

Solutes

The requirement of purity of medical compound used in an injection often makes it necessary to take special purification of chemical grade used. The best chemical grade to be used but further purification may be necessary. Factors to be consider for the quality of solute:

i. Purity
ii. Freedom for toxicity
iii. Freedom from contamination (microbial and pyrogen contamination)
iv. Solubility of compound
v. Freedom from gross dirt.

Added Substances

The USP includes in this category all substances added to a parenteral preparation to improve or safeguard its quality. An added substance may:

i. Effect solubility, as does sodium benzoate in caffeine and sodium benzoate injection.

ii. Provide patient comfort, as do substances added to make a solution isotonic or near physiological pH.

iii. Enhance the chemical stability of a solution, as do antioxidants, Inert gases, chelating agents and buffers.

iv. They may preserve the preparation against microbial growth.

Antimicrobial Agents

i. The USP states that antimicrobial agents in bacteriostatic or fungistatic concentrations must be added to preparations contained in multiple-dose containers.

ii. They must be present in adequate concentration at the time of use to prevent the multiplication of microorganisms inadvertently introduced into the preparation while withdrawing a portion of the contents with a hypodermic needle and syringe.

The USP provides a test for antimicrobial preservative effectiveness to determine that an antimicrobial substance or combination adequately inhibits the growth of microorganisms in a parenteral product (Table 11.2). Compatability studies of the microbial agents should be performed before using them into the formulation.

Buffers

Buffers are used primarily to stabilize a solution against pH, which result in to reduction in the chemical degradation that might occur if the pH changes. Buffer systems employed should normally have low buffering capacity as if buffering capacity of product is high it may disturb significantly the body's

Table 11.2: Preservative used and their concentration

Preservative	Typical concentration (%)
Benzyl alcohol	1–2
Chlorbutanol	0.5
Methylparaben	0.1–0.18
Propylparaben	0.01–0.02
Phenol	0.2–0.5
Thiomersal	<0.01

buffering systems when injected. In addition, the buffer range and effect on the activity of the product must be evaluated carefully (Table 11.3).

Table 11.3: Buffers used in parenteral products

Buffer	pH range
Acetate	3.8–5.8
Ammonium	8.25–10.25
Ascorbate	3.0–5.0
Benzoate	6.0–7.0
Bicarbonate	4.0–11.0
Citrate	2.1–6.2
Diethanolamine	8.0–10.0
Glycine	8.8–10.8
Lactate	2.0–4.1
Phosphate	3.0–8.0
Succinate	3.2–6.6
Tartrate	2.0–5.3
Tromethamine (TRIS. THAM)	7.1–9.1

A parenteral product should be formulated with a pH close to physiological, unless stability or solubility considerations preclude this. Often, the pH selected for the product is a compromise between the pH of maximum stability, solubility, and physiological acceptability.

Antioxidants

Antioxidants are required to preserve products because of the ease with which many drugs are oxidized. Antioxidants are included in parenteral formulations, although their use is now in decline, and EU guidelines discourage their use unless no other alternative exists. A preferred method of preventing oxidation is simply to exclude oxygen; this is usually achieved by purging the product with nitrogen and creating a nitrogen headspace within the container. Where this process is insufficient:

i. A metal chelator, such as disodium edentate (0.05%)
ii. An antioxidant compound, such as ascorbic acid or sodium metabisulfite (1%, and 0.3%, respectively).

Tonicity agents are used in many parenteral and ophthalmic products to adjust the tonicity. However, not all preparations need to be isotonic. The agents most commonly used are electrolytes and mono- or disaccharides.

Pyrogen

"Microbial pyrogen" as opposed to "gram-negative bacterial endotoxin" has become a general descriptive term for many substances. However, some gram-negative bacteria, mycobacteria fungi and also some viruses can produce pyrogenic substances, but the pyrogens produced by gram-negative bacteria, i.e. the endotoxins, are of significance to the pharmaceutical industry.

Bacterial **endotoxins,** found in the outer membrane of gram-negative bacteria are members of a class of phospholoipids called lipopolysaccharides (LPS). LPS are not exogenous products of gram-negative bacteria. The release of LPS from bacteria takes place after death and lysis of the cell. Good examples of pyrogen producing gram-negative bacteria are *Escherichia coli, Proteus, Pseudomonas, Enterobacter* and *Klebsiella*.

Sources: There are several sources of pyrogens in parenteral and medical device products. Usual sources are: the water used as the solvent or in the processing; packaging components; the chemicals, raw materials or equipment used in the preparation of the product. Good practices include the control of microbiological contamination and endotoxin levels of contamination in the potential sources mentioned above. Additionally, if the drug substance is biological, the incomplete process of removal of the microorganism during purification can result in high endotoxin levels.

Control: General processing procedures for physical components of parenteral products, such as stoppers and vials provide for washing these components with pyrogen-free water prior to sterilization. Another source of endotoxin is WFI— water for injection. Generally ambient temperature WFI systems present the greatest problems. Remember—endotoxins result from high levels of microorganisms and are not removed by sterilizing or filtration. It is difficult to remove endotoxins from products once present. It is better to keep products and components relatively endotoxin-free than to have to remove them once present. The most common depyrogenation procedures for physical components include incineration and removal by washing (also called dilution). Distillation has been shown to be effective and the most reliable method in removing endotoxin from contaminated water samples. For physical components, such as stoppers and tubing, rinsing or dilution with pyrogen-free water systems is most common. Historically, glass components are rinsed with pyrogen-free water and dry heat sterilized at high temperatures. There are other methods used for chemical components and manufacturing equipment. Pyrogen testing is discussed latter in this chapter.

Method of Preparing Parenteral Suspension and Solution

Two basic methods are used to prepare parenteral suspension or solution.

Method 1

Step 1: Aseptically combining sterile powder and vehicle.

Step 2: This method involves dispersing or dissolving sterile milled active ingredients into sterile vehicle system. (Solvents + necessary excipients).

Step 3: Aseptically milling the resulting suspension as required.

Step 4: Aseptically filling the milled suspension or solution in to suitable containers.

For example, this process is used to prepare penicillin G suspension (Fig. 11.5).

Method 2

In-situ formation of parenteral suspension:

Step 1: *In-situ* crystal formation by combining sterile solutions (Fig. 11.6).

Step 2: In this method active ingredients are dissolved in suitable solvent system.

Step 3: A sterile vehicle system or counter solvent is added to step 2 solution that causes active ingredient to crystallize.

Step 4: The organic solvent is aseptically removed the resulting suspension is aseptically milled as necessary and then filled in suitable container.

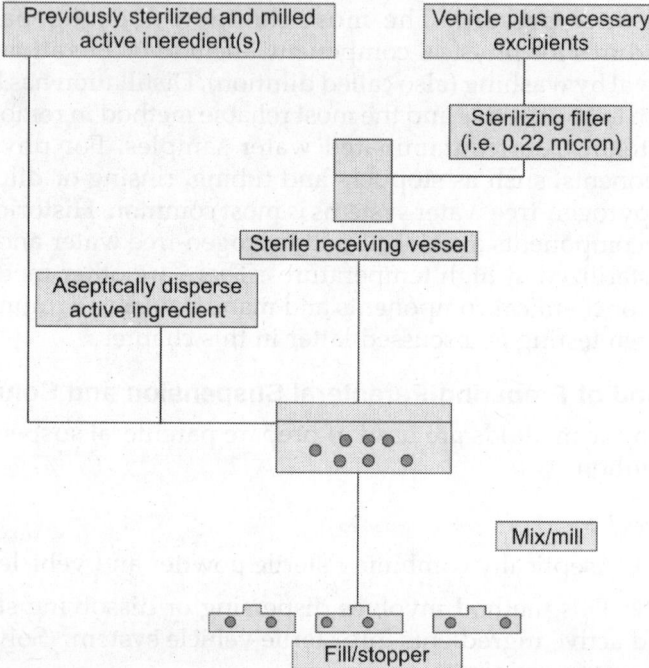

Fig. 11.5: Method 1 of preparing parenteral suspension and solution

For example, testerone in parenteral insulin suspension (Fig. 11.6).

TOTAL PARENTERAL NUTRITION

Nutrition is an important factor to aid patient to full recovery. Total parenteral nutrition is a method of supplying nutrients to the body by an intravenous route. It is indicated to patients with impaired or non functional gastrointestinal tract. The aim of administering TPN are to improve the nutritional status of the patient, to attain weight gain and to enhance the healing process.

Total parenteral nutrition (PN) is the feeding of a person intravenously, bypassing the usual process of eating and digestion. The person receives nutritional formulae that contain nutrients, such as glucose, salts, amino acids, lipids and added vitamins and dietary minerals. It is called **total parenteral nutrition (TPN)** or **total nutrient admixture (TNA)** when no

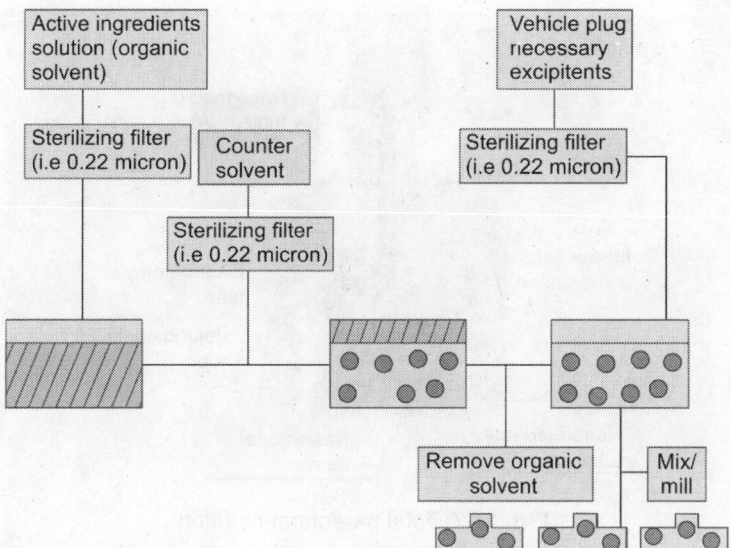

Fig. 11.6: Method 2 of preparing parenteral suspension

significant nutrition is obtained by other routes, and **partial parenteral nutrition (PPN)** when nutrition is also partially enteric. It may be called **peripheral parenteral nutrition (PPN)** when administered through vein access in a limb rather than through a central vein as **central venous nutrition (CVN)** (Fig.11.7).

There are three methods of giving TPN:

  i. Peripheral: When the TPN is less hypertonic and given through peripheral vein.

 ii. Atrial: TPN is given by inserting atrial catheters.

iii. Central: When TPN is given for long-term intravenous therapy and catheter is inserted in subclavian vein.

Components of TPN

Prepared solutions generally consist of water and electrolytes; glucose, amino acids, and lipids; essential vitamins, minerals and trace elements are added or given separately. Previously lipid emulsions were given separately but it is becoming more common for a "three-in-one" solution of glucose, proteins, and lipids to be administered (Fig. 11.7).

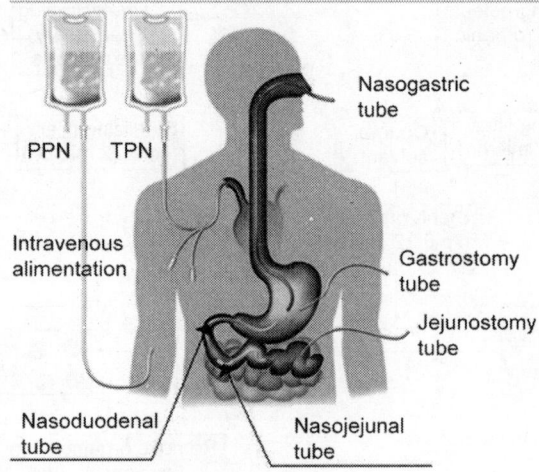

Fig: 11.7: Total parenteral nutrition

TPN are commercially prepared by pharmacist in aseptic conditions and they generally contains:

    i. Dextrose
   ii. Amino acids
  iii. Electrolytes
   iv. Vitamins
    v. Minerals
   vi. Fat.

The TPN solutions are prepared depending upon the:

    i. Energy requirement of patient
   ii. Protein requirement of patient
  iii. Fluid requirement and tolerance of patient
   iv. Fat requirement of patient
    v. Dextrose requirement of patient
   vi. Type of electrolytes required by the patient.

Duration

Short term TPN may be used if a person's digestive system has shut down, e.g. peritonitis, and they are at a low enough weight to cause concerns about nutrition during an extended hospital stay. Long-term PN is occasionally used to treat people suffering from accident, surgery, or digestive disorder.

Complications

TPN fully bypasses the GI tract and normal methods of nutrient absorption. Possible complications, which may be significant, are listed below.

Infection: TPN requires a chronic IV access for the solution to run through, and the most common complication is infection of this catheter.

Blood clots: Chronic IV access leaves a foreign body in the vascular system, and blood clots on this IV line are common.

Fatty liver and liver failure: Fatty liver is usually a more long-term complication of TPN the pathogenesis is due to using linoleic acid (an omega-6 fatty acid component of soybean oil) as a major source of calories.

Hunger: Because patients are being fed intravenously, the subject does not physically eat, resulting in intense hunger pangs. The brain uses signals from the mouth (taste and smell), the stomach/GI tract (fullness) and blood (nutrient levels) to determine conscious feelings of hunger.

Pregnancy: Pregnancy can cause major complications when trying to properly dose the nutrient mixture. Because all of the baby's nourishment comes from the mother's bloodstream, the doctor must properly calculate the dosage of nutrients to meet both recipient's needs and have them in usable forms.

Side Effects of TPN

1. Development of mouth sores
2. Poor night vision
3. Changes in skin quality
4. Weight loss
5. Fever
6. Stomach pain.

DIALYSIS

Dialysis is the process of removing waste products and excess fluid from the body. Dialysis is necessary when the kidneys are not able to adequately filter the blood. Dialysis allows patients with **kidney failure** a chance to live productive lives. Dialysis works on the principles of the diffusion of solutes and ultrafiltration of fluid across a semi-permeable membrane. Diffusion is a property of substances in water; substances in water tend to move from an area of high concentration to an area of low concentration. Blood flows by one side of a semi-permeable membrane, and a dialysate, or special dialysis fluid, flows by the opposite side.

There are two types of dialysis:
  i. Hemodialysis
  ii. Peritoneal dialysis.

Hemodialysis removes wastes and water by circulating blood outside the body through an external filter, called a dialyzer, that contains a semipermeable membrane. The blood flows in one direction and the dialysate flows in the opposite. The counter-current flow of the blood and dialysate maximizes the concentration gradient of solutes between the blood and dialysate, which helps to remove more urea and creatinine from the blood. The dialysis solution has levels of minerals like potassium and calcium that are similar to their natural concentration in healthy blood. For another solute, bicarbonate, dialysis solution level is set at a slightly higher level than in normal blood, to encourage diffusion of bicarbonate into the blood, to act as a pH buffer to neutralize the metabolic acidosis that is often present in these patients. The levels of the components of dialysate are typically prescribed by a nephrologist according to the needs of the individual patient (Fig. 11.8).

In **peritoneal dialysis**, wastes and water are removed from the blood inside the body using the peritoneum as a natural semipermeable membrane. Wastes and excess water move from the blood, across the peritoneal membrane and into a special dialysis solution, called dialysate, in the abdominal cavity (Fig. 11.9).

In peritoneal dialysis, a sterile solution containing glucose (called dialysate) is run through a tube into the peritoneal cavity, the abdominal body cavity around the intestine, where the peritoneal membrane acts as a partially permeable membrane.

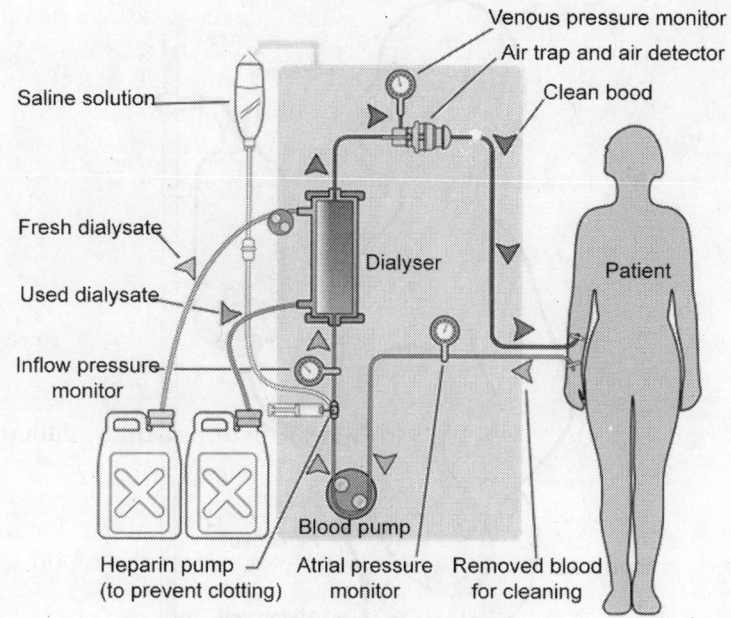

Fig 11.8: Haemodialysis

This exchange is repeated 4–5 times per day; automatic systems can run more frequent exchange cycles overnight. Peritoneal dialysis is less efficient than hemodialysis, but because it is carried out for a longer period of time the net effect in terms of removal of waste products and of salt and water are similar to hemodialysis. Peritoneal dialysis is carried out at home by the patient, often without help. This frees patients from the routine of having to go to a dialysis clinic on a fixed schedule multiple times per week. Peritoneal dialysis can be performed with little to no specialized equipment (other than bags of fresh dialysate).

Advantages and Disadvantages of Kidney Transplants Compared with Dialysis

Advantages

The patients can return to a normal lifestyle—dialysis may require a lengthy session in hospital, 3 times a week, leaving the patient very tired after each session.

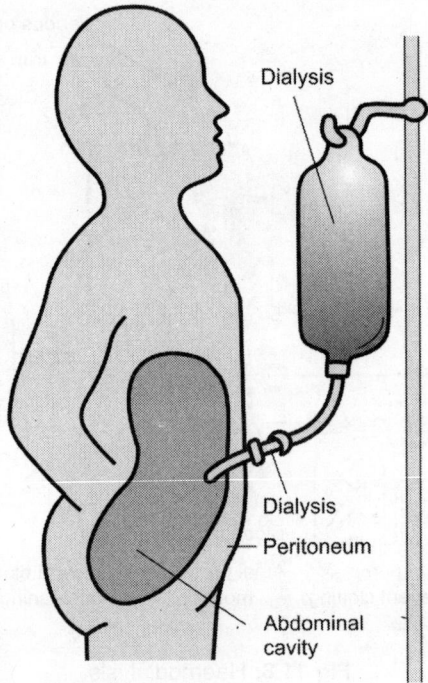

Fig 11.9: Schematic diagram of peritoneal dialysis

  i. A dialysis machine will be available for other patients to use.

  ii. Dialysis machines are expensive to buy and maintain.

Disadvantages

Transplants require a suitable donor—with a good tissue match. The donor may be a dead person, or a close living relative who is prepared to donate a healthy kidney, we can survive with one kidney.

  i. The operation is very expensive.

  ii. There is a risk of rejection of the donate kidney—immunosuppressive drugs have to be used.

  iii. Transplantation is not accepted by some religions.

STERILITY TESTING FOR PARENTERAL PREPARATIONS
1. Pyrogen test
2. Test for particulate matter
   i. Light obstruction particle count test
   ii. Microscopic particle count test
3. Test for sterility of ophthalmic products
4. Leak test (already discussed)

Test for Pyrogens

It is used to check for the presence of pyrogens in the parenteral formulation. Two general tests are performed.
   i. Rabbit test
   ii. LALs test

Rabbit Test

The pyrogen test is designed to limit to an acceptable level the risks of febrile reaction in the patient to the administration, by injection, of the product concerned. Unless otherwise specified in the individual monograph, inject into an ear vein of each of three rabbits 10 ml of the test solution per kg of body weight, completing each injection within 10 minutes after start of administration. The test solution is either the product, constituted if necessary as directed in the labeling, or the material under test treated as directed in the individual monograph and injected in the dose specified therein. Assure that all test solutions are protected from contamination. Perform the injection after warming the test solution to a temperature of 37 ± 2°. Record the temperature at 30-minute intervals between 1 and 3 hours subsequent to the injection.

Test Interpretation

Consider any temperature decreases as zero rise. If no rabbit shows an individual rise in temperature of 0.5° or more above its respective control temperature, the product meets the requirements for the absence of pyrogens. If any rabbit shows an individual temperature rise of 0.5° or more, continue the test using five other rabbits. If not more than three of the eight rabbits show individual rises in temperature of 0.5° or more and if the sum of the eight individual maximum temperature rises does not exceed 3.3°, the material under examination meets the requirements for the absence of pyrogens.

LALs test: Limulus amebocyte lysate (LAL) is an aqueous extract of blood cells (amoebocytes) from the horseshoe crab, limulus polyphemus. LAL reacts with bacterial endotoxin or lipopolysaccharide (LPS), which is a membrane component of gram-negative bacteria. This reaction is the basis of the LAL test.

Method: Blood is removed from the horseshoe Crab's pericardium and the blood cells are separated from the serum using centrifugation and are then placed in distilled water, which causes them to swell up and burst ("lyse"). This releases the chemicals from the inside of the cell (the "lysate"), which is then purified and freeze-dried. To test a sample for endotoxins, it is mixed with lysate and water; endotoxins are present if coagulation occurs.

Particulate Evaluation

Parenteral solutions should be essentially free from particulate matter which can be observed on visual inspection. This test describes the physical tests performed to enumerate extraneous particles with specific size ranges. Particulate matter includes mobile, randomly sourced, extraneous substances, other than gas bubbles that cannot quantified by chemical analysis due to less amount and of their heterogeneous compositions.

Methods

   i. Light obscuration method
   ii. Microscopic method.

Light obscuration Method

This method applies for ophthalmic solution including solutions constituting form sterile solids, for which the test for particulate matter is specified in the individual monograph.

The parenteral product meets the requirements of the test if the average numbers of particles present in the units tested does not exceed the appropriate value listed in the following Table 11.4.

Table 11.4: Light obscuration particle count test

	Diameter	
	≥ 10 µm	≥ 25 µm
SVI	6000	600/container
LVI	25	3/ml

If the average number of particles exceeds this limit, the test article is subjected to microscopic method.

Microscopic Method

This method is performed when some particles are not exactly detected by the light obscuration method. This test enumerates the subvisible particles essentially solid, particulate matter present in the parenteral preparation. The test sample is collected on a microporous membrane filter.

The USP injection meets the requirements of the test if the average number of particles present in the units tested does not exceed the appropriate value listed in the following Table 11.5.

Table 11.5: Microscopic method particle count test

	Diameter	
	≥ 10	≥ 25
SVI	3000	300/container
LVI	12	2/ml

Sterility Test

This is used to test the presence of microorganisms in the test solution. It is done by 2 methods.

  i. Membrane filtration method

 ii. Direct inoculation (immersion) method.

Membrane filtration method: In this the test solution is first passed through assize exclusion membrane capable of retaining the microorganisms. The concept is that the microorganisms will collect on the surface of a 0.45 micron pore size filter. The filter is rinsed and then the membrane is transferred to appropriate test medium as specified in the monograph.

Direct inoculation (immersion) method: In this the test article is directly inoculated into the test medium and then the medium is incubated for the growth of microorganisms, if present.

Test media: The test media are fluid thioglycollate medium (FTM) and soybean casein digest medium (SCDM). FTM is selected based upon its ability to support the growth of anaerobic and aerobic microorganisms. SCDM is selected based upon its ability to support a wide range of aerobic bacteria and fungi (i.e. yeasts and molds).

Incubation time: In both the methods the test medium after the transferring of the test solution is to be incubated for 3 days in case of bacteria and 5 days in case of fungi and then the growth is compared with that of standard. If no growth is observed then the sample passes the test and it meets the GMP requirements.

The following Table 11.6 outlines the requirement for sterility testing as per USP. The requirement for sterility testing as per USP.

Table 11.6: The requirement for sterility testing as per USP

Volume/container	Minimum quantity to test in each media
< 1 ml	The entire contents of each container
1–40 ml	Half the contents of each container but not < 1 ml
41–100 ml	20 ml
> 100 ml	10% of the contents of the container, but not < 20 ml

PACKAGING, LABELLING AND STORAGE OF INJECTIONS

Containers for injections, including closures, must not interact physically and chemically with the preparation.

   i. **Single-dose container:** A single dose container is a hermetic container holding a quantity of sterile drug intended for parenteral administration as a single dose, and which when opened cannot be re-sealed with assurance that sterility has been maintained.

  ii. **Multiple-dose container:** A multiple-dose container is a hermetic container that permits withdrawal of successive portions of the contents without changing the strengths, quality, or purity of the remaining portion.

The Labels on Containers of Parenteral Products Must State

1. The name of the preparation.
2. For liquid preparation, the percentage content of the drug or amount of the drug; for dry preparation—the amount of the active ingredient present and the volume of liquid to be added to the dry preparation to prepare a solution or suspensions.
3. The route of administration.
4. Statement of storage conditions and expiration.
5. The name of the manufacturer and distributor.
6. The identifying lot number.

PRACTICE QUESTIONS

1. Define the term parenteral products. Give their advantages and disadvantages.
2. Give classification of parenteral products with the help of suitable examples, based on their route of administration.
3. Give classification of parenteral products with the help of suitable examples on the basis of their injection volumes.
4. Discuss in brief the various factors which can effect solubility of parenteral drugs?
5. Write in detail about the various components of parenteral formulation.
6. Name some common apparatus used for the production of water for injections.
7. Write short notes on:
   a. Non aqueous vehicles used for parenteral
   b. Specification for purified water
   c. Water miscible vehicles
   d. Solutes
8. Write short notes on (Reference to parenteral products):
   a. Antimicrobial agents
   b. Preservatives

c. Buffers

d. Antioxidant

9. Describe in detail about the various types of containers used for parenteral formulation.

10. What are the desired characteristics of parenteral container?

11. Write in brief about rubber closure and their criteria of selection for parenteral products.

12. Write in brief about the test done for parenteral closures.

13. Describe the methods used for preparation of parenteral suspension.

14. Describe the methods used for preparation for parenteral solution.

15. Enlist various important operations involved during formulation of parenteral preparation.

16. Give the classification of various methods of sterilization for parenteral products.

17. Write short notes on:

a. Packaging of parenteral

b. Labelling of parenteral

18. What is lyophilization? Give basics of lyophilization.

19. Enumerate various factors affecting efficiency of lyophilization.

20. Describe the evaluation test done for parenteral formulations.

OBJECTIVE TYPE QUESTIONS

1. .... dosage forms of drugs are injected directly into body tissue through one or more layer of skin and mucous

2. The US Pharmacopeia (USP) defines Small volume parenteral (SVPs) which contains .... and Large-volume parenterals (LVPs) containing ....

3. .... is the removal of water from frozen material. It is an excellent method for preserving microbes and heat-sensitive materials, such as proteins, plasma, etc.

4. The two USP tests for determining glass types are .... and ....

5. Match the following

S.No	Parenteral dosage form	Route of administration
1.	Intradermal	A. Inside an eye
2.	Subcutaneous	B. Into the skin
3.	Intravitreal	C. Under the skin
4.	Intracavernous	D. Into the epidural space of the spinal cord
5.	Intrathecal	E. Into the base of the penis
6.	Epidural	F. Through the theca of the spinal cord
7.	Intraosseous infusion	G. Into the bone marrow
8.	Intravenous	H. Into the peritoneum
9.	Intra-articular	I. Within a vein
10.	Intraperitoneal	J. With in joints

6. Match the following

S.No	Type of glass	Material used
1.	Type I Glass	A. Treated soda lime glass
2.	Type II Glass	B. Ordinary soda lime glass
3.	Type III Glass	C. Untreated soda lime glass
4.	Type NP Glass	D. Highly resistant borosilicate glass

7. Which of the following is the evaluation tests for parenteral preparations:

a. Pyrogen test and test for particulate matter

b. Light obstruction particle count test and microscopic particle count test

c. Test for sterility of ophthalmic products and powder attack test

d. a and b

e. All of the above

Answers

1. Parenteral

2. Less than 100 ml, more than 100 ml

3. Lyophilization (freeze drying)

4. Powdered glass test, water attack test

5. 1. B, 2. C, 3. A, 4. E, 5. F, 6. D, 7. G, 8. I, 9. J, 10. H

6. 1. D, 2. A, 3. C, 4. B

7. d

Chapter 12

Ophthalmic Products

Eye is unique and very precious organ. It is considered as window of the soul. We can enjoy and viewed the whole world only with this organ. There are many eye ailments which affect this organ and one can loss the eyesight also. Therefore, many ophthalmic drug delivery systems are available. These are classified as conventional and newer drug delivery systems. Most commonly available ophthalmic preparations are eye-drops and ointments. But, these preparations when in-stilled into the cul-de-sac are rapidly drained away from the ocular cavity due to tear flow and lachrymal nasal drainage. Only a small amount is available for its therapeutic effect resulting in frequent dosing. Thus inefficient drug delivery into the eye occurs due to rapid tear turnover, lachrymal drainage and drug dilution by tears.

Topical administration for ocular therapeutics is ideal because of smaller doses required compared to the systemic use, its rapid onset of action and freedom from systemic toxicity Topically applied ocular drugs have to reach the inner parts of the eye and transcorneal penetration is believed to be the major route for drug absorption. Corneal absorption is much slower process than elimination. For many drugs K loss (first order elimination rate) is approximately 0.5–0.7 min and K absorption (first order absorption rate) is about 0.001/min. The sum of these two rate constants control the fraction of the applied dose absorbed into the eye. So, the ocular bioavailability can be increased by decreasing K loss or by increasing K absorption. The former can be achieved by modifying the ocular dosage forms and the latter by formulating ocular dosage forms containing lipophilic prodrugs or by adding penetration enhancers. Therefore to optimize topical ocular drug delivery system prolonged contact time with the corneal surface and better penetration through cornea is necessary. A considerable amount of effort has been made in ophthalmic drug delivery since 1970's. The two main approaches attempted are improvement in bioavailability and controlled release drug delivery.

PHYSIOLOGY OF EYE

The eyeball has three regions namely outermost core which comprises of transparent cornea and white opaque sclera, middle which contains iris anteriorly, the choroids and the ciliary body posteriorly and the last layer contains retina which is an extension of central nervous system. Ophthalmic preparations are generally act at cornea and this region acts as the gateway for these formulations. The penetration of drugs through the cornea is dependent on the stroma epithelium of the cornea. This layer is of lipid bilayer, i.e. fat–water–fat structure and thus control passage of drugs. The aqueous humor and the vitreous humor constitute fluid systems in the eye. This fluid escapes through the posterior part and anterior part (Fig. 12.1).

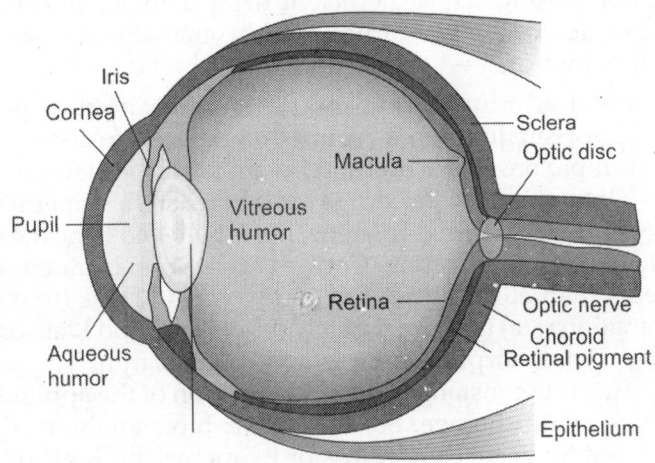

Fig. 12.1: Physiology of eye

The ocular drugs applied topically are intended for the local action or for penetration into the anterior chamber and thus distributes to whole tissues of the eye. Some of the characters required for optimizing the ocular drug delivery system are:

- Good corneal penetration
- Prolong contact time with corneal tissue
- Simplicity of instillation for the patient
- Sterility of the product
- Non irritative and comfortable form (viscous solution should not provoke lachrymal secretion and reflex blinking)
- Appropriate rheological properties and concentrations of the viscous system.

Ideal Ophthalmic Formulations

- Ophthalmic solutions should be free from foreign particles
- Insoluble drug particles are made in the form of suspensions. They should be redispersed on shaking the container.
- There should not be any leakage from the finished dosage form of ointment and it should be free from larger particles and it must meet the requirements of metal particles.

For achieving the drug delivery through the eye, different methods were followed like:

1. Using different grades of polymers
2. Preparation of viscous gels
3. Colloidal preparations
4. Using erodible and non erodible inserts which prolong the drug retention time at cornea.

It is found that the cornea offers more resistance to the negatively charged compounds.

Various Types of Ophthalmic Products

Ophthalmic products include:

1. Eyedrops
2. Eye-lotions
3. Contact lens solution
4. Eye ointments

1. **Eyedrops:** These are the aqueous or oily solutions or suspensions that are instilled into the conjuctival sac of the

eye. These are used as anaesthetics, anti-inflammatory agents, antiseptics, diagnostic agents, mitotics, mydriatics and artificial tears, e.g. atropine sulphate eyedrops BPC, hyoscine eyedrops BPC, physostigmine eyedrops BPC requirements for an Ideal eyedrops product:

i. Should be sterile in condition

ii. Absence of foreign particles

iii. They should not cause any pain and irritation.

Ophthalmic solutions are the most common dosage form for delivering the drug to the eye. As it is solution all the ingredients are completely soluble and there is almost no physical inference with the eyesight. The disadvantage of these solutions is the contact time of drug is less with the absorbing tissue. Efforts have been made to improve this contact time by including the viscosity enhancing agents but their use is restricted to low viscosities only because the drops can be dispensed through the eyedroppers and to minimize the blurring the vision. Generally, the viscous solutions produce residue on eyelashes and around eye if they are spilled during dispensing. It can be easily removed by wiping with most cloth to closed eye.

2. **Eye-lotions:** These are the aqueous solutions that are used in undiluted condition for bathing the eye in first aid or in home, e.g. sodium chloride eye-lotion.

3. **Contact lens solutions:** These are the aqueous solutions intended for lubricating, cleaning and hydrating contact lenses, e.g. thimerosal contact lens solution.

4. **Eye ointments:** These are placed in the conjunctival sac or applied to the margins of the eyelids, e.g. bacitracin ophthalmic ointment.

Conclusion

An ideal system should have effective drug concentration at the target tissue for a tended period of time with minimum systemic effect. Patient acceptance is very important for the design of any comfortable ophthalmic drug delivery system. Major improvements are required in each system like improvement in sustained drug release, large scale manufacturing and stability. Combination of drug delivery systems could open a new directive for improving the therapeutic response of a non-efficacious system. They can overcome the limitations and combine the advantages of different systems.

ISOLATED KEY POINTS

- Most commonly available ophthalmic preparations are eye-drops and ointments.
- The eyeball has three regions namely outermost core which comprises of transparent cornea and white opaque scelra, middle which contains iris anteriorly, the choroids and the cilliary body posteriorly and the last layer contains retina which is an extension of central nervous system.
- Ophthalmic preparations are generally act at cornea and this region acts as the gateway for these formulations. The penetration of drugs through the cornea is dependent on the stroma epithelium of the cornea. This layer is of lipid bilayer, i.e. fat–water–fat structure and thus control passage of drugs.
- **Various types of ophthalmic products are:**
  i. Eyedrops
  ii. Eye-lotions
  iii. Contact lens solution
  iv. Eye ointments
- **Eyedrops:** These are the aqueous or oily solutions or suspensions that are instilled into the conjuctival sac of the eye. These are used as anaesthetics, anti-inflammatory agents, antiseptics, e.g. atropine sulphate eyedrops BPC.
- **Eye-lotions:** These are the aqueous solutions that are used in undiluted condition for bathing the eye in first aid or in home, e.g. sodium chloride eye-lotion.
- **Contact lens solutions:** These are the aqueous solutions intended for lubricating, cleaning and hydrating contact lenses, e.g. thimerosal contact lens solution.
- **Eye ointments:** These are placed in the conjunctival sac or applied to the margins of the eyelids, e.g. bacitracin ophthalmic ointment.

PRACTICE QUESTIONS

1. What are ophthalmic products? What should be the characteristics of an idea ophthalmic product?

2. Give physiology of eye with the help of a heat and labeled diagram.

3. Enlist the various types of ophthalmic products, give their examples.

4. How ophthalmic products bioavailability can be increase by controlled drug delivery system?

5. What are the recent advancement in ophthalmic products? Give their examples.

6. What are the various test employed for ophthalmic solutions?

OBJECTIVE TYPE QUESTIONS

1. Ophthalmic preparations are generally act at ....which acts as the gateway for these formulations

2. Soft contact lenses are made up of the most widely used material ....

3. The desired particle size of the suspension for the preparation of ophthalmic preparation is ....

4. To check for the presence of pyrogens in the ophthalmic formulation the two general tests done are ....

5. LAL stands for............... and it is an aqueous extract of blood cells (amoebocytes) from ....

6. Pyrogens are............ they are .... in nature, which is a membrane component of gram ......bacteria

7. Which of the following is not the characters required for optimizing the ocular drug delivery system:
   a. Good corneal penetration
   b. Prolong contact time with corneal tissue
   c. Hypertonicity of the solution
   d. Sterility of the product

8. Which of the following is not an ophthalmic product:
   a. Specs and sunglasses
   b. Eye-lotions
   c. Contact lens solution
   d. Eye ointments

9. Which of the following are the evaluation tests for ophthalmic preparations.
   a. Particle size determination and test for clarity of ophthalmic solutions
   b. Test for pH of the solution and test for particulate matter
   c. Test for sterility of ophthalmic products and pyrogen test
   d. All of the above

Answers

1. Cornea
2. Poly-2-hydrosyethylmethacrylate
3. 5–10 µm or less
4. Rabbit test and LALs test
5. Limulus amebocyte lysate, horseshoe crab, Limulus polyphemus.
6. Bacterial endotoxin, lipopolysaccharide, negative
7. c
8. a
9. d

Chapter 13

Experiments in Pharmaceutics

Object: To prepare and submit 20 ml of cresol with soap solution IP (Lysol solution).

Principle: Solutions are liquid preparations that contain one or more soluble chemical substances dissolved in liquid solvents. Solutions are generally prepared by four methods:

  a. By simple solution.

  b. By chemical reactions.

  c. By simple solution with sterilization.

  d. By extraction.

Solution is a mixture of two compounds namely solute and solvent. Solute is the smaller component present in the solution and is usually non-volatile in nature. Solvent is the larger component present and is also known as vehicle. Most of the drugs are non-polar or semi polar. Hence, they cannot be easily solubilized in water. Therefore, special methods are used to prepare solutions. Solubility can be enhanced by using co-solvents (examples are glycerin, ethyl alcohol, propylene glycol) or complexation (example is a combination of iodine and potassium iodide) or surfactants (example is cresol with soap solution). Solutions are usually used for their specific therapeutic effect of solute either internally or externally. To increase the shelf-life and aesthetic value of solutions, various additives are also added, such as stabilizers, preservatives, colouring agents, flavouring agents, and sweetening agents. Solutions form most of the dosage forms like mixtures, enemas, mouthwashes, gargles, eardrops, eyedrops, etc.

Cresol is a mixture of O, m and p-cresol. It acts as disinfectant. The solubility of cresol in water is only about 3% whereas the quantity of cresol present in this preparation is 50%. To dissolve this much quantity of cresol, a solubilising agent is required. Vegetable oil contains free fatty acids, which react with potassium hydroxide and form soap. This soap acts as solubilising agent. The vegetable oil may be cottonseed, linseed, soybean or similar oils, which have a saponification value not greater than 205 and an iodine value, not less than 100. Solubilization is a process which allows a poorly water-soluble solute to go into solution and hence increases the solubility of the materials. It requires the presence of surface-active agents, which form colloidal aggregates when added in higher concentrations. The concentration of the surfactant at which the micelle formation takes place called the critical micelle concentration or CMC. The poorly soluble material either dissolves or gets absorbed onto the micelle at CMC, which ultimately increase the solubility of the material.

Observation Table

S. No	Ingredients	Quantity given	Quantity taken
1.	Cresol	500 ml	10 ml
2.	Vegetable oil	180 g	3.6 g
3.	Potassium hydroxide	42 g	0.84 g
4.	Purified water (q.s)	1000 ml	20 ml

Procedure: Dissolve the potassium hydroxide in 250 ml of purified water, add the vegetable oil and heat on a water bath, mixing thoroughly, continue to heat until a small portion dissolves in water without separation of oily drops. Add the cresol, mix thoroughly and add sufficient purified water to produce the required volume.

Category: Disinfectant.

Storage: Store in cool and dry place, keep away from the children.

Direction: For external use only as a general disinfectant. It is unsuitable for use on human beings.

Uses: Lysol (cresol with soap) solution is a phenolic compound used as a disinfectant for domestic or hospital use like disinfection of floors, bathrooms, washbasins, organic waste, such as sputum, faeces, urine, etc.

Precautions

1. Not to be used in the vicinity of infants, such as nursery, children wards, etc.
2. Not to be used in places where food is prepared and served.

EXPERIMENT 2

Object: To prepare and submit 20 ml of strong iodine solution IP.

Principle: Strong iodine solution contains 10% w/v of iodine (limits 9.5 to 10.5) and 6.0% w/v of potassium iodide. KI (limits 5.7 to 6.3). Iodine with potassium iodide forms compounds called poly iodides. The higher poly iodides are more soluble than lower ones. Hence a rapid solution of the iodine is affected by using the potassium iodide in concentrated solution. Alcohol in the preparation is used as a menstruum. Another advantage of alcohol is that it quickly evaporates when the solution is applied over the skin leaving behind the iodine in very fine particle size. Due to this a larger surface area of iodine comes in contact with the body, which results in quicker absorption. It also dissolves cutaneous fat and hastens penetration and absorption and provides some additional antibacterial effect. The preparation is used as a topical antiseptic agent. The preparation cannot be applied to azwounds and abrasions because the alcohol in the tincture is very irritating to open tissues. The preparation is stored in a well-closed container because alcohol and iodine are volatile in nature. The iodine stains the skin, clothes and vessels made from porcelain and metal, therefore, it should be stored only in glass containers. The iodine stain can be removed by sodium thiosulphate solution.

Observation Table

S. No	Ingredients	Quantity given	Quantity taken
1.	Iodine	100 g	2 g
2.	Potassium iodide	60 g	1.2 g
3.	Purified water	100 ml	2 ml
4.	Alcohol (90%) sufficient to produce	1000 ml	20 ml

Procedure: First dissolve the potassium iodide in little volume of water. Dissolve the iodine in above solution; add sufficient alcohol 90% to produce the required volume.

Category: Antiseptic

Storage: Store in a well-closed container, the materials of which are resistant to iodine.

Direction: For external use only.

Uses: Strong iodine is used to treat overactive thyroid, iodine deficiency, and to protect the thyroid gland from the effects of radiation from radioactive forms of iodine.

EXPERIMENT 3

Object: To prepare and submit 20 ml of weak iodine solution IP (tincture iodine).

Principle: Weak iodine solution is used internally in hypothyroidism and externally as antiseptic to treat wounds. In this preparation the concentration of iodine required is 20 mg/ml. As this preparation is used internally as well as externally alcohol 50% (absolute alcohol 50 ml + water 50 ml) is used as a vehicle. Iodine is very slightly soluble in water. Its solubility can be increased using potassium iodide. Potassium iodide reacts with iodine to form polyiodides that are more soluble in alcohol 50%

$$Kl + nl_2 \, Kl \, l_2 + Kl \, 2l_2 + Kl \, 3l_2 + \rightarrow + Kl \, nl_2$$
Polyiodides

Polyiodides are more soluble in water by ion induced dipolar interaction. Alcohol is used in this preparation because of two reasons; (a) When this preparation is applied to the wounds, alcohol precipitates the proteins and forms a protective layer, (b) alcohol absorbs heat from the body and gets evaporated thereby causing cooling effect. Since iodine (present in iodine solution) reacts with some ingredients of ordinary glass container, iodine resistant container like amber coloured container is used to store iodine solutions.

Observation Table

S. No	Ingredients	Quantity given	Quantity taken
1.	Iodine	20 g	0.4 g
2.	Potassium iodide	25 g	0.5 g
3.	Alcohol (50%) (q.s)	1000 ml	20 ml

Procedure: Dissolve the potassium iodide and iodine in sufficient alcohol 50% to produce the required volume.

Category: Antiseptic, iodine supplement in hypothyroidism.

Storage: Store in a well-closed container, the materials of which are resistant to iodine.

Direction: For external use only.

Uses: As a disinfectant.

EXPERIMENT 4

Object: To prepare and submit 20 ml of strong ammonium acetate solution IP.

Principle: This preparation contains 57.5% w/v of ammonium acetate and it is prepared by reacting glacial acetic acid with ammonium bicarbonate and strong solution of ammonia.

$$NH_4HCO_3 + CH_3COOH \rightarrow CH_3COONH_4 + H_2O + CO_2$$
$$CH_3COOH + NH_4HCO_3 \rightarrow CH_3COONH_4 + H_2O + CO_2$$

A large open vessel is used to allow easy escape of the carbon dioxide and avoid spillage due to frothing. It is not possible to prepare the solution by reacting glacial acetic acid with ammonium bicarbonate alone, because the reaction between these substances ceases before the formation of required amount of ammonium acetate. As more and more ammonium acetate is going to form, concentration of acetate ions is going to increase and ionization of CH_3COOH is going to decrease and ultimately is will stop. Ammonium hydroxide is used to neutralize the unreacted acid and to make the preparation alkaline with pH range 7.6 to 8.1. The pH is adjusted by using two indicators, i.e. bromothymol blue and thymol blue. They give different colourations at different pH. Blue and yellow colours are obtained only in pH range 7.6 to 8.1. Bromothymol blue checks the lower limit, i.e. pH 7.6 and thymol blue checks the upper limit, i.e. pH 8.1. Bromothymol blue changes colour as follows:

Yellow → pH 6.0 green → pH 7.6 blue → pH 14

Thymol blue changes colour as follows:

Red → pH 2.1 → yellow → pH 8.1 →

green → pH 9.2 → violet → pH 14

The preparation is stored in lead free glass containers because ammonium acetate dissolves lead salts readily and due to extraction of lead from the glass, the preparation will become toxic and can cause lead poisoning. Diaphoretic mixture is used to lower the raised body temperature by increasing the excretions of body fluids in the form of sweat and urine.

Observation Table

S. No	Ingredients	Quantity given	Quantity taken
1.	Glacial acetic acid.	453 g	
2.	Ammonium bicarbonate	470 g	
3.	Ammonium solution strong	100 ml	
4.	Purified water (q.s)	1000 ml	20 ml

Note: Glacial acetic acid Wt/ml 1.047–1.052 g

Procedure: Mix the glacial acetic acid with about 350 ml the purified water, add the ammonium bicarbonate in small quantities, at a time and stir until it is completely dissolved. Add sufficient quantity of ammonia solution until one drop of the resulting solution, diluted with 10 drops of water, gives a full blue colour with 1 drop of bromothymol blue, and a full yellow with thymol blue. Add sufficient purified water to produce the required volume.

Category: Bactericidal.

Storage: Store in a well-closed lead free glass container.

Direction: For external use only.

Uses: As a bactericide.

EXPERIMENT 5

Object: To prepare 100 ml of Lugol's solution (IP), label it and dispense it in a suitable container.

Theory: Lugol's solution contains 5% w/v of iodine and 10% w/v of potassium iodide. Iodine is poorly soluble in water. Iodine with potassium iodide forms a compound called polyiodide.

$$I_2 + KI \rightarrow KI.I_2/KI.2I_2/KI.3I_2/KI.4I_2$$

The higher polyiodides are more soluble than the lower polyiodides potassium iodide may be replaced by sodium iodide.

Materials: Measuring cylinder, beaker and glass rod.

Reagents: Iodine, potassium iodide, distilled water.

Formula

S. No	Ingredients	Quantity given	Quantity taken
1.	Iodine	50 g	5 g
2.	Potassium iodide	100 g	10 g
3.	Distilled water (q.s)	1000 ml	100 ml

Calculation

1. 1000 ml of water contain 50 g of iodine

   Hence 100 ml of water contains $= \dfrac{50 \times 100}{1000} = 5\,g$

2. 1000 ml of water contain 100 g of potassium iodide

   Hence 100 ml of water contains $= \dfrac{100 \times 100}{1000} = 10\,g$

Procedure

1. Dissolved potassium iodide in minimum quantity of water.
2. Add iodine, shake well until the solution is clear.

3. Finally make up the volume with distilled water.

4. Transfer it into the bottle and label and dispense it.

Category: As a preservative and germicidal.

Storage: Store in a well-closed iodine resistant container and *"Keep it in a cool and dry place"*.

Uses

1. As a source of iodine.

2. As a germicide.

3. As a preservative.

4. Used in hyperthyroidism.

EXPERIMENT 6

Object: To prepare 100 ml of strong ammonium acetate solution (IP), label it and dispense it in a suitable container.

Theory: Strong ammonium acetate solution contain 57.5% w/v of ammonium acetate. Acetic acid and ammonium bicarbonate is reacted to form ammonium acetate as shown below

$$NH_4HCO_3 + CH_3COOH \rightarrow CH_3COONH_4 + H_2O + CO_2$$

After this reaction all acid is not neutralized. To neutralize it strong ammonia solution is added drop wise.

$$CH_3COOH + NH_3 \rightarrow CH_3COONH_4$$

pH of this solution is maintained by using bromothymol blue and thymol blue.

Materials: Measuring cylinder, beaker and glass rod.

Reagents: Ammonium bicarbonate, glacial acetic acid, ammonia solution, distilled water.

Formula

S. No	Ingredients	Quantity given	Quantity taken
1.	Glacial acetic acid	453 ml	45.3 ml
2.	Ammonium bicarbonate	470 g	47 g
3.	Ammonia solution	100 ml	10 ml
4.	Distilled water (q.s)	1000 ml	100 ml

Calculation

1. 1000 ml of water contain 453 ml of glacial acetic acid

   Hence 100 ml of water contains $= \dfrac{453 \times 100}{1000} = 45.3$ ml

2. 1000 ml of water contain 470 g of ammonium bicarbonate

   Hence 100 ml of water contains $= \dfrac{470 \times 100}{1000} = 47$ g

3. 1000 ml of water contain 100 ml of ammonia solution

   Hence 100 ml of water contains $= \dfrac{100 \times 100}{1000} = 10$ ml

Procedure

1. Mix glacial acetic acid with small amount of water, add ammonium bicarbonate to dissolve it.
2. Add sufficient amount of ammonia solution to neutralize the resulting solution.
3. One drop of resulting solution diluted with 10 drops of water, gives full blue colour with a drop of bromothymol blue solution and a full yellow colour with one drop of thymol blue solution. (pH 8.0 to 9.6).
4. Finally add sufficient quantity of water to make up the volume.
5. Transfer it into the bottle label and dispense it.

   Category: As a diaphoretic.

   Storage: Store in a well-closed container free from lead. *"Keep it in a cool and dry Place"*.

Uses

1. Used as diuretic (diuretics are those substances which causes urination, they also help in hypertension as they causes elimination of sodium ions).
2. As a diaphoretic (diaphoretic are those substances which lower the elevated body temperature by causing sweating and urination).

EXPERIMENT 7

Object: To prepare and submit 100 ml of aluminium hydroxide antacid suspension.

Principle: Suspensions are disperse systems in which finely divided insoluble solid drug particles are dispersed in a suitable liquid vehicle. The solid particles are known as dispersed phase whereas liquid vehicle is known as continuous phase. A good suspension should have the following characteristics:

1. Finely divided solid particles should not settle rapidly and should be readily re-dispersed on gentle shaking of the container, if particles settle.
2. The suspension should be easily removed from the container.
3. The suspended particles should not form hard cake.
4. The suspension should have optimum viscosity, which facilitates the easy removal from the container and easily spread on the body surface.
5. The suspension should be free from gritty particles.

Suspension should be packed in suitable containers. For less viscous preparations use narrow mouthed bottles and, wide mouth bottles for thick preparations.

Based on the nature of the solids present suspensions can be classified as follows:

a. Flocculated suspensions, e.g. tetanus toxoid suspension
b. Deflocculated suspensions, e.g. procaine penicillin G suspension.

Aluminium hydroxide gel is an antacid suspension. It is also known as aluminium hydroxide suspension or aluminium hydroxide mixture. It is colloidal suspension, hence does not required the use of suspending agent because of the strong affinity that exists between the dispersed phase aluminium hydroxide and water. As a result there is increase in viscosity and aluminium hydroxide gel gets easily dispersed in water.

Aqueous aluminium hydroxide antacid suspension tends to thicken as gel during shelf-life. This gelling accelerated during storage under warm conditions (30–40°C). This problem can be circumvented by the addition of sorbitol in concentration from 0.5–7% depending on the concentration of aluminium hydroxide in suspension. Aluminium hydroxide has constipating effect; therefore, it is normally combined with magnesium hydroxide, which provides laxative effect in commercial antacid formulations.

The taste of an antacid must be considered for consumers' acceptance. Sorbitol imparts a cool sweet pleasant taste. The parabens are used as preservatives. Peppermint oil as flavouring agent. Alcohol serves as vehicle. Amaranth solution is added to impart colour to the preparation.

Observation Table

S. No	Ingredients	Quantity given	Quantity taken
1.	Aluminium hydroxide gel dried	360 g	36 g
2.	Sorbitol	70 ml	7 ml
3.	Sodium saccharine	0.5 g	0.05 g
4.	Methyl paraben	2 g	0.2 g
5.	Propyl paraben	0.2 g	0.02 g
6.	Peppermint oil	0.05 ml	0.005 ml
7.	Alcohol	10 ml	1 ml
8.	Amaranth solution	q.s	q.s
9.	Purified water	q.s to 1000 ml	q.s to 100 ml

Procedure: Dissolve methyl paraben, propyl paraben, sodium saccharine, and peppermint oil in alcohol in clean dry vessel. In another beaker take nearly one-half of volume of purified water and add sorbital solution. Mix well. To this solution add the alcoholic solution and stir well. Add Aluminium hydroxide in small proportions with continuous stirring. Add amaranth solution and mix. The entire product may be passed through a colloidal mill or homogeniser. Transfer to a measuring cylinder, add sufficient purified water to produce required volume. Mix well. Transfer to suitable bottle.

Category: Antacid suspension

Storage: Store in a cool and dry place, away from sunlight.

Direction: Shake well before use.

Use: As antacid in peptic ulcers and hyperchlorhydria.

EXPERIMENT 8

Object: To prepare and submit 20 ml of liquid paraffin emulsion IP.

Principle: Emulsions are defined as disperse systems consisting of two immiscible liquids, one of which is distributed through the other in the form of minute globules, the system being stabilized by adding the third substance, the emulsifying agent. Emulsions are of two types:

1. Oil in water (o/w), in which the oil is dispersed in the water continuous phase. These emulsions are preferred for internal use. In these emulsions gum acacia, tragacanth and soaps of monovaslent bases like Na^+, NH_4^+, K^+ are used as emulsifying agents.

2. Water in oil (w/o), in which the water is dispersed in the oil, the continuous phase. In these emulsions wool fat, resins, bees wax and soaps of divalent bases like Ca^{++}, Mg^{++}, Zn^{++} are used as emulsifying agents.

Emulsions are prepared by different methods. They are dry gum method, wet gum method and bottle method.

While preparing the acacia emulsions for extemporaneous use, primary emulsion formula must be used. Based on the nature of the oil different formulas are there.

Nature of oil	Examples	Ratios of ingredients		
		Oil	Water	Acacia gum
Fixed oil	Castor oil	4	2	1
Mineral oil	Liquid paraffin	3	2	1
Volatile oil	Turpentine oil	2	2	1
Oleo gum resin	Male fern extract	1	2	1

Liquid paraffin emulsion is oil in water emulsion, made by the dry gum method, containing 50% v/v of liquid paraffin (limits 45.0–55.0). Liquid paraffin constitutes oil phase and purified water constitutes water phase.

Acacia is used as an emulsifying agent, which forms oil in water type of emulsion. Tragacanth is used as an emulsifying agent as well as viscosity-increasing agent, which stabilize the o/w acacia emulsion. Sodium benzoate is used as the preservative, especially for the oil phase. It prevents the surface growth of the microorganisms when emulsion is packed. High vapour pressure of chloroform allows it to concentrate on the surface of the emulsion and also fill the empty area of the bottle, which will not allow any growth of microorganisms on the surface of the mixture.

Observation Table

S. No	Ingredients	Quantity given	Quantity taken
1.	Liquid paraffin	500 ml	10 ml
2.	Indian gum, in powder form	125 g	2.5 g
3.	Tragacanth, in powder form	5 g	0.1 g
4.	Sodium benzoate	5 g	0.1 g
5.	Vanillin	0.5 g	0.01 g
6.	Chloroform	2.5 ml	0.05 ml
7.	Glycerin	125 ml	2.5 ml
8.	Purified water, sufficient to produce	1000 ml	20 ml

Procedure: Triturate liquid paraffin and the chloroform with the Indian gum, the tragacanth and vanillin. Add in one quantity 250 ml of purified water and triturate until a creamy emulsion formed. Add the glycerin and the sodium benzoate dissolved in 50 ml of purified water. Add sufficient purified water to produce 1000 ml. Mix.

Category: Laxative.

Storage: Store in a well-closed container; Protected from light.

Direction: Shake well before use.

Uses: It is used as laxative in chronic constipation and also used during pregnancy for the emptying of faecal material in body before surgery.

EXPERIMENT 9

Object: To prepare and submit 20 ml of castor oil emulsion.

Principle: Castor oil is a fixed oil and is not miscible with water. To make it miscible a third substance known as emulsifying agent in the ratio of 4:2:1, i.e. oil, water, gum will be used for the preparation of primary emulsion. Gum acacia will be used as emulsifying agent because emulsions prepared with gum acacia remain stable for sufficient long-time.

Observation Table

S. No	Ingredients	Quantity given	Quantity taken
1.	Castor oil	8 ml	5.33 ml
2.	Water	30 ml	20 ml

Procedure: By *Wet gum method:*

Thoroughly clean and dry a pestle and mortar. Weigh out 2 g gum acacia and transfer it to the mortar. Measure 4 ml water and triturate it with gum so as to form mucilage. To this add 8 ml castor oil in small quantities at a time with thorough trituration after each addition. Triturate briskly without ceasing until a clicking sound is produced and the product becomes white or nearly white. At this stage the emulsion is known as primary emulsion. Add about 10 ml more of vehicle in small quantities at a time with constant trituration so as to get a homogeneous product.

Transfer the emulsion to a measure, add more of vehicle to produce the final volume 30 ml, stir thoroughly so as to form a uniform emulsion. Transfer the preparation to a bottle, cork, polish the bottle to remove fingerprints, label and dispense.

Direction: Shake well before use.

Category: Purgative.

Storage: Store in a well-closed container, protected from light.

Uses: As a purgative for the free evacuation of especially causing evacuation of the bowels.

Precautions: Because of its prompt action castor oil should not be administered at bedtime, preferably it should be given early in the morning.

EXPERIMENT 10

Object: To prepare and submit 20 ml of cod liver oil emulsion IP.

Principle: Cod liver oil is fixed oil obtained from the fresh liver of the cod fish. This emulsion is given in case of the deficiency of vitamin A and D as an anti-rachitic. The emulsion should be protected from light to prevent the degradation of vitamin A.

The emulsion is prepared by the dry gum method. Acacia is the emulsifying agent and tragacanth is the emulsion stabilizer. Saccharin sodium is used as the sweetening agent. Benzaldehyde spirit is used as the flavouring agent and chloroform is used as the preservative.

Observation Table

S. No	Ingredients	Quantity given	Quantity taken
1.	Cod liver oil	500 ml	10 ml
2.	Acacia, in powder form	125 g	2.5 g
3.	Tragacanth, in powder form	7.5 g	0.15 g
4.	Benzaldehyde spirit	2.5 ml	0.05 ml
5.	Saccharin sodium	1 g	0.02 g
6.	Chloroform	2.5 ml	0.05 ml
7.	Purified water (q.s)	1000 ml	20 ml

Procedure: Take the cod liver oil in dry mortar and disperse acacia powder and tragacanth powder in it. Add the required volume of water, as for the primary emulsion formula, all at once to the mortar and triturate in one direction only until primary emulsion is formed. Dilute carefully, transfer to a measure, add the saccharin sodium solution, benzaldehyde spirit and chloroform with constant stirring and make up the volume with purified water.

Category: Source of vitamin A and D (Anti-rachitic).

Storage: Store in a well-closed container in a cool place.

Direction: Shake well before use.

Uses: As a nutritional supplement. Since, it is obtained from fish oils, it has high levels of the omega 3 fatty acids, EPA and DHA.

Is also a source of vitamin A and vitamin D.

EXPERIMENT 11

Object: To prepare 100 ml of methyl salicylate liniment (BP), label and dispense it in a suitable container.

Theory: Liniments are liquid and semi liquid preparations meant for application to the skin. Liniments are usually applied to the skin with friction and rubbing of the skin. The liniments may be alcoholic or oily solutions or emulsions. Alcohol helps in the penetration of medicaments into the skin and also increases its counter irritant or rubifacient action. Arachis oil is used in some liniments, which spread more easily on the skin. Generally liniments contain medicaments possessing analgesic, rubifacient, and smoothing, counter irritant or stimulating properties. A liniment should not be applied to broken skin because it may cause excessive irritation. Methyl salicylate is water insoluble compound, so we use arachis oil to dissolve it.

Materials: Measuring cylinder, beaker, pipette, glass rod.

Reagents: Methyl salicylate, arachis oil.

Formula

S. No	Ingredients	Quantity given	Quantity taken
1.	Methyl salicylate	250 ml	25 ml
2.	Arachis oil (q.s)	1000 ml	100 ml

Calculation

1. 1000 ml of arachis oil contain 250 ml of methyl salicylate

Hence 100 ml of arachis oil contains $= \dfrac{250 \times 100}{1000} = 25$ ml

Procedure

1. Take a small quantity of arachis oil in a beaker.
2. Add required amount of methyl salicylate.
3. Shaken well so, that methyl salicylate gets mixed with arachis oil.
4. Finally add required amount of arachis oil to make up the volume.
5. Transfer it into the bottle, label and dispense it in a suitable container.

Category: Anti-inflammatory agent.

Storage: Store in a well-closed container, keep it in a cool and dry place.

Uses

1. Used as an analgesic (which relieves in pain).
2. As an anti-inflammatory agent (which reduces inflammation).

EXPERIMENT 12

Object: To prepare 100 ml of turpentine liniment (BP), label it and dispense it in a suitable container.

Theory: Liniments are liquid or semi liquids preparations meant for external application that are intended to be applied to the unbroken skin with friction. They contain substances possessing analgesic, rubifacient, soothing or stimulating properties. Liniments are usually applied to the skin with friction. Liniments should be dispensing in colour-fluted bottles in order to distinguish from preparation meant for internal use.

Turpentine oil is the volatile oil and has the action of counter irritant and rubifacient. This preparation is an emulsion type of liniment, which contains turpentine oil as oil phase and water as aqueous phase. Here soft soap is used as an emulsifying agent to form oil in water type of emulsion.

Materials: Measuring cylinder, beaker, mortar and pestle, glass rod.

Reagents: Soft soap, camphor, turpentine oil, distilled water.

Formula

S. No	Ingredients	Quantity given	Quantity taken
1.	Soft soap	90 g	9 g
2.	Camphor	50 g	5 g
3.	Turpentine oil	650 ml	65 ml
4.	Distilled water	1000 ml	100 ml

Calculation

1. 1000 ml of water contain 90 g of soft soap

Hence 100 ml of water contains $= \dfrac{90 \times 100}{1000} = 9\,g$

2. 1000 ml of water contain 50 g of camphor.

Hence 100 ml of water contains $= \dfrac{50 \times 100}{1000} = 5\,g$

3. 1000 ml of water contain 650 ml of turpentine oil.

Hence 100 ml of water contains $= \dfrac{650 \times 100}{1000} = 65\,ml$

Procedure

1. Dissolve the soft soap in water and make a smooth solution of camphor in turpentine oil.

2. Gradually add turpentine oil solution to soft soap solution with continuous stirring to form a thick creamy emulsion.

3. Finally add sufficient amount of water to make up the volume.

4. Transfer it into the bottle, label and dispense it.

Category: As a counter irritant and rubefacient.

Storage: Store in a well-closed container away from light.

Uses

1. Used as a counter irritant.

2. Used in myalgia, sprain, and fibrositis.

EXPERIMENT 13

Object: To prepare and submit 20 ml of chloramphenicol eye-drop.

Principle: Eyedrops are aqueous or oily solutions or suspensions for instillation into the eye. They should be sterile and prepared under conditions appropriate for the preparation of sterile products (aseptic conditions). The method of sterilization is stated in each monograph. For aqueous solutions, water for injection should be used.

Eyedrops should be prepared in a vehicle which is bactericidal and fungicidal. They should be isotonic with lachrymal secretions (which is equivalent to 0.9% NS).

Dropper plastic bottles are suitable for packing eyedrops. Label should instruct the patient to discard the unused eyedrops no longer than one month after opening the container.

The following care is to be taken while preparing the eyedrop first of all it is to be sterilize by heating at 98 to 100°C for 30 minutes. It is to be store in airtight containers, below 25°C and used within three months and it should be protected from light.

Observation Table

S. No	Ingredients	Quantity given	Quantity taken
1.	Benzalkonium chloride solution	0.02 ml	0.004 ml
2.	Disodium edetate	50 mg	10 mg
3.	Sodium chloride	900 mg	180 mg
4.	Water for injection q.s	100 ml	20 ml

Category: Eyedrop

Storage: Store in a cool and dry place, away from sunlight.

Direction: Keep out of the reach of children always close the stopper after use.

Use: As a wide spectrum antibiotic used for the treatment of acute bacterial infection of the external eye.

EXPERIMENT 14

Object: To prepare and submit 20 ml of benzalkonium chloride solution.

Principle: Eyedrops are aqueous or oily solutions or suspensions for instillation into the eye. They should be sterile and prepared under conditions appropriate for the preparation of sterile products (aseptic conditions). The method of sterilization is stated in each monograph. For aqueous solutions, water for injection should be used.

Eyedrops should be prepared in a vehicle which is bactericidal and fungicidal. They should be isotonic with lachrymal secretions (which is equivalent to 0.9% NS).

Dropper plastic bottles are suitable for packing eyedrops. Label should instruct the patient to discard the unused eyedrops no longer than one month after opening the container.

The following care is to be taken while preparing the eyedrop first of all it is to be sterilize by heating at 98 to 100°C for 30 minutes. It is to be store in airtight containers, below 25°C and used within three months and it should be protected from light.

Observation Table

S. No	Ingredients	Quantity given	Quantity taken
1.	Benzalkonium chloride solution	0.02 ml	0.004 ml
2.	Disodium edetate	50 mg	10 mg
3.	Sodium chloride	900 mg	180 mg
4.	Water for injection q.s	100 ml	20 ml

Procedure

1. Mix benzalkonium chloride solution, disodium edetate and sodium chloride in about 2/3 the amount of vehicle (water for injection).

2. Transfer to a cylinder and complete to volume with water for injection.

3. Transfer into a suitable container and fix a red label.

Category: Eyedrop

Storage: Store in a cool and dry place, away from sunlight.

Direction: Keep out of the reach of children, always close the stopper after use.

Use: As an antiseptic with bactericidal and bacteriostatic activities

EXPERIMENT 15

Object: To prepare and submit 20 ml of potassium chlorate gargles.

Principle: Generally, gargles are used to relieve soreness in mid throat infections and most have a deodorant effect. A bactericide, e.g. phenol or thymol. It is usually present but not in high enough concentration for significant antibacterial activity; however, it may exert a mild anesthetic effect. Potassium chlorate is included in gargles for its weak astringent effect on superficial cells, which helps to remove the tone of a relaxed throat; it also stimulates the flow of saliva, which relives dryness. The best-known gargles are phenol garlic, potassium chlorate and phenol garlic and thymol glycerin compound.

Observation Table

S. No	Ingredients	Quantity given	Quantity taken
1.	Potassium chlorate	30 g	0.6 g
2.	Liquid phenol	15 ml	0.3 g
3.	Water q.s	1000 ml	20 ml

Procedure: Dissolve the weighed amount of potassium chlorate is about 15 ml of water. To this add liquefied phenol and add sufficient water to produce the required volume. Transfer to a container, label and dispense. The secondary label "for external use only" must be attached.

Category: Antibacterial.

Storage: Store in a cool and dry place, away from children.

Direction: These gargles should be diluted with ten times its volume of warm water before use.

Uses: These gargles are used at sialogogue and astringent. Potassium chlorate is a sialogogue (which increases the flow of saliva) and astringent (which precipitate the proteins).

EXPERIMENT 16

Object: To prepare and submit 20 ml of antiseptic mouthwash.

Principle: Mouthwashes are aqueous solutions with pleasant taste and odour used to clean deodorize the buccal cavity. They are very refreshing, particularly to bedridden patients. Generally, they contain antibacterial agents, alcohol, glycerin, sweetening agents and flavouring agents. In this preparation thymol and borax used as antibacterial agents, alcohol as solvent, glycerin as sweetening agent, sodium bicarbonate can dissolve mucous.

Observation Table

S. No	Ingredients	Quantity given	Quantity taken
1.	Thymol	0.3 g	0.006 g
2.	Alcohol	35 ml	0.7 ml
3.	Borax	20 g	0.4 g
4.	Sodium bicarbonate	10 g	0.2 g
5.	Glycerin	80 ml	1.6 ml
6.	Flavour	Adequate	Adequate
7.	Water q.s	1000 ml	20 ml

Procedure: Dissolve the required quantity of thymol in alcohol. In another beaker dissolve borax and sodium bicarbonate in water and mix the both solutions. Add glycerin and sufficient quantity of flavour mix well. Add the water to produce required volume.

Category: Antibacterial.

Storage: Store in a cool and dry place, away from children.

Direction: 'Dilute with an equal volume of warm water before use'. 'Not to be swallowed in large quantities'.

Uses: To enhance oral hygiene.

Mouthwash has antiseptic and antiplaque effect it also kills the bacterial which causes plague, gingivitis and bed breath.

EXPERIMENT 17

Object: To prepare 100 ml of chloroform spirit (IP), label and dispense it in a suitable container.

Theory: Spirits are alcoholic or hydroalcoholic preparations containing volatile substances. The volatile ingredient may be in the form of solid, liquid or gas. They are generally used for internal as well as externally as inhalations for their medicinal value while there major use is as flavouring agent. They may be used in the formulation of aromatic waters or as pharmaceutical aids.

Spirits are prepared by following methods:

1. Simple solution
2. Solution with maceration
3. Chemical reaction
4. Distillation

Materials: Measuring cylinder, beaker, amber coloured bottle, glass rod.

Reagents: Chloroform, alcohol (90%).

Formula

S. No	Ingredients	Quantity given	Quantity taken
1.	Chloroform	50 ml	5 ml
2.	Acohol 90% (q.s)	1000 ml	100 ml

Calculation

1000 ml of alcohol contain 50 ml of chloroform

Hence 100 ml of alcohol contains $= \dfrac{50 \times 100}{1000} = 5 \, ml$

Procedure

1. Take a little quantity of alcohol in measuring cylinder.
2. Add required quantity of chloroform.
3. Shake well so, that chloroform get mixed with alcohol.
4. Add more amount of alcohol to make up the volume.
5. Transfer it into the bottle, label and dispense it.

Category: Pharmaceutical aid

Storage: Store in a well-closed air tight container, away from sunlight.

Uses

1. As a pharmaceutical aid.
2. As a sweetening agent.
3. As a preservative.
4. Also used as a main ingredient of carminative mixture.

EXPERIMENT 18

Object: To prepare 100 ml of calamine lotion (IP), label it and dispense it in a suitable container.

Theory: These are liquid preparation, meant for external application without friction. Lotion may be used for local application, such as cooling, soothing and protective purpose. They are generally applied for antiseptic action. Alcohol is sometimes included in aqueous lotion for its cooling and soothing effect. Calamine is a combination of zinc carbonate mixed with ferric oxide, which gives pink colour to it. Zinc oxide has got astringent, protective and antiseptic action. Bentonite (colloidal hydrated aluminium silicate) is used for its suspending property. It helps to suspending the insoluble calamine in distilled water. Sodium citrate acts as deflocculating agent or peptizing agent, i.e. prevents the lotion from being too viscous, it also act as a buffer and maintain the pH appropriate to skin. Liquid phenol is an antiseptic as well as preservative. Glycerin acts as an emollient (smoothening effect) and as an humectant (prevents the loss of moisture from the skin).

Material required: Mortar and pastel, beaker, measuring cylinder, glass rod, and bottle.

Reagents: Calamine, zinc oxide, bentonite, sodium citrate, glycerin, liquefied phenol, lavender oil, distilled water.

Formula

S. No	Ingredients	Quantity given	Quantity taken
1.	Calamine	150 g	15 g
2.	Zinc oxide	50 g	5 g
3.	Bentonite	30 g	3 g
4.	Sodium citrate	5 g	0.5 g
5.	Liquid phenol	5 ml	0.5 ml
6.	Glycerin	50 ml	5 m
7.	Lavender oil	1 ml	10.01 ml
8.	Distilled water (q.s)	1000 ml	100 ml

Calculation

1. 1000 ml of water contain 150 g of calamine.

Hence 100 ml of water contains $= \dfrac{150 \times 100}{1000} = 15\,g$

2. 1000 ml of water contain 50 g of zinc oxide.

Hence 100 ml of water contains $= \dfrac{50 \times 100}{1000} = 5\,g$

3. 1000 ml of water contain 30 g of bentonite.

Hence 100 ml of water contains $= \dfrac{30 \times 100}{1000} = 3\,g$

4. 1000 ml of water contain 5 g of sodium citrate.

Hence 100 ml of water contains $= \dfrac{5 \times 100}{1000} = 0.5\,g$

5. 1000 ml of water contain 5 ml of liquified phenol.

Hence 100 ml of water contains $= \dfrac{5 \times 100}{1000} = 0.5\,ml$

6. 1000 ml of water contain 50 ml of glycerin.

Hence 100 ml of water contains $= \dfrac{50 \times 100}{1000} = 5$ ml

7. 1000 ml of water contain 1 ml of lavender oil.

Hence 100 ml of water contains $= \dfrac{1 \times 100}{1000} = 0.01$ ml

Procedure

1. Weigh the required amount of calamine, zinc oxide and bentonite.
2. Transfer it in a mortar and add a small quantity of water to make a cream.
3. Add required amount of liquid phenol.
4. Dissolve sodium citrate in small quantity of water and mix with above mixture.
5. Add required amount of glycerol and two drops of lavender oil.
6. Finally add water to make up the volume.
7. Transfer it to a bottle, label it and dispense it in a suitable container.

Category: As a protective.

Storage: "Store in a well-closed container". "Keep it in a cool and dry place".

Uses

1. It is used to remove roughness of skin.
2. Meant for external application without friction.

EXPERIMENT 19

Object: To prepare and submit 20 g of non-staining iodine ointment BPC.

Principle: Non-staining iodine ointment BPC is used as a counter-irritant. The fixed oils and many fats obtained from vegetable and animal sources contain unsaturated constituents. The iodine combines with double bonds of the unsaturated constituents. Hence free iodine is not available.

$$CH_3 (CH_2)_7 CH = CH - (CH_2)_7 COOH + I_2 \rightarrow$$

Oleic acid $\quad CH_3 (CH_2)_7 CHI = CHI (CH_2)_7 COOH$

Di-iodo stearic acid

If complete iodine is not combined then the free iodine gives brown colour to the product and leaves a stain when applied. In other words, if complete iodine is combined with unsaturated oils and fats, then the final ointment attains greenish black colour. It leaves no stain when rubbed onto the skin. Hence, they are known as non-staining iodine ointments. Iodine is easily soluble in unsaturated oils like arachis oil. To enhance the rate of solubilization, powdered form of iodine is preferred. Iodine solution is heated to complete the reaction between iodine and arachis oil. Heating must be done at not more than 50°C, because at high temperatures iodine sublimes.

Methyl salicylate is volatile in nature. To avoid evaporation of methyl salicylate, it is added when the preparation is at lower temperature. Stirring should be done slowly to prevent air entrapment when the preparation starts thickening. Iodine acts as a counter irritant. Methyl salicylate also serves as a counter irritant and a flavouring agent. Yellow soft paraffin is used as a base. This is a semisolid preparation. Some quantity of preparation will go waste during manufacture of semisolids. 2 g extra is calculated to nullify loss during manufacture of 20 g non-staining iodine ointment, i.e. quantities of ingredients are calculated for 22 g.

Observation Table

S. No	Ingredients	Quantity given	Quantity taken
1.	Methyl salicylate	50 ml	1 ml
2.	Iodine	50 g	1 g
3.	Arachis oil	150 g	3 g
4.	Yellow soft paraffin q.s	1000 g	20 g

Procedure: Depending on the quantity of preparation to be submitted, the working formula is calculated.

1. Iodine is dissolved in arachis oil at room temperature by simple stirring in a beaker.

2. Heat the above solution on water bath at 50°C with occasional stirring until the brown colour disappears (or greenish black colour appears).

3. Sufficient quantity of yellow soft paraffin is added (previously heated to 40°C), stirred slowly, cooled to solidify.

4. When the above preparation is at semi-liquid consistency, methyl salicylate is added, stirred slowly, allowed for complete solidification.

5. The ointment is transferred to a tightly-closed wide-mouthed container.

6. The container is capped, polished, labelled, and submitted.

Composition: Each g contains 47.5 to 52.5 mg of iodine.

Category: Counter irritant.

Storage: Store in a cool place.

Directions: For external use only, do not apply on broken skin.

Uses: The deeply penetrating action of ointment provides long-lasting relief from backaches, waist pains, muscle strains, and sprains.

EXPERIMENT 20

Object: To prepare and submit 25 gm of non-staining iodine ointment BPC.

Principle: Ointments are semisolid preparations for application to the skin or mucosa. The common property of semisolid preparation is the ability to cling to the surface of application for reasonable duration before they are washed. This adhesion is due to their plastic rheological behaviour, which allows the semisolid pharmaceutical preparations are pastes, creams, gel, etc. Ointments are semisolid greasy preparations for application to the skin, rectum and nasal mucosa. The base is usually anhydrous and contains the medicament in solution or suspension form. They are used for their emollient effect on skin, for the protection of lesion and for topical medication.

Ointment bases: Apart from drug, ointment consists of ointment base. Various types of bases are used depending upon characteristic of drug and product required. The bases are classified as:

1. Oleaginous bases, e.g. soft paraffin, hard paraffin, etc.
2. Absorption bases, e.g. non-emulsified w/o, etc.
3. Water removable (miscible).
4. Water soluble.

Ointment base used in non-staining iodine ointment is yellow soft paraffin, which is an example of oleaginous base. Yellow soft paraffin is preferred for darker constituent.

Non-staining iodine ointment which is used as analgesic, anti-inflammatory contain iodine which is complex with fixed oil containing fatty acid at 60°C which result in colour change from brown to green black. This is done because free iodine has staining property and is irritant to skin and is used for veterinary use only. Here paraffin, i.e. ointment base is only used as a carrier of drug. Paraffin can absorb only 2% of iodine but fixed oil can bind with iodine equivalent to its weight.

Equation

$$CH_3 (CH_2)_7 CH = CH (CH_2)_7 COOH + I_2 \rightarrow$$

Oleic acid　　　　　$CH_3 (CH_2)_7 CHI-CHI(CH_2)_7 COOH$

di-iodo-stearic acid

Observation Table

S. No	Ingredients	Quantity given	Quantity taken
1.	Iodine	50 g	1.25 g
2.	Arachise oil	150 ml	3.75 ml
3.	Methyl salicylate	50 g	1.25 g
4.	Yellow soft paraffin q.s	1000 g	25 g

Procedure: Finely powder the iodine in a glass mortar and add required amount to the oil taken in a glass stoppered conical flask and stir well. Heat at 50°C and stir occasionally until the brown colour has changed to greenish black. Take the required quantity of yellow soft paraffin in a china dish and warm soft paraffin and mix well. Measure the required volume of methyl salicylate and mix with base containing the iodized oil. Then pour into a warm wide mouth light resistance glass container and allow cooling without further stirring.

Category: Counter-irritant, rubifacient, and anti-inflammatory and analgesic.

Storage: Store in cool place and protect from light. Keep container tightly closed after use.

Direction: For external use only. Not to be applied on broken skin. Apply to affected area with rubbing.

Uses: Used as a anti-inflammatory and analgesic.

EXPERIMENT 21

Object: To prepare 10 gm of coal tar and salicylic acid ointment.

Principle: Ointments are semisolid preparations for application to the skin or mucosa. The common property of semisolid preparation is the ability to cling to the surface of application for reasonable duration before they are washed. This adhesion is due to their plastic rheological behaviour, which allows the semisolid pharmaceutical preparations are pastes, creams, gel, etc. Ointments are semisolid greasy preparations for application to the skin, rectum and nasal mucosa. The base is usually anhydrous and contains the medicament in solution or suspension form. They are used for their emollient effect on skin, for the protection of lesion and for topical medication.

Ointment bases: Apart from drug, ointment consists of ointment base. Various types of bases are used depending upon characteristic of drug and product required. The bases are classified as:

1. Oleaginous bases, e.g. soft paraffin, hard paraffin, etc.

2. Absorption bases, e.g. non-emulsified w/o, etc.

3. Water removable (miscible).

4. Water soluble.

Ointment base used in non-staining iodine ointment is yellow soft paraffin, which is an example of oleaginous base. Yellow soft paraffin is preferred for darker constituent.

Observation Table

S. No	Ingredients	Quantity given	Quantity taken
1.	Coal tar	20 g	0.20 g
2.	Polysorbate 80	40 ml	0.40 ml
3.	Salicylic acid	20 g	0.20 g
4.	Emulsifying wax	114 g	1.14 g
5.	White soft paraffin	190 g	1.9 g
6.	Coconut oil	540 ml	5.40 ml
7.	Liquid paraffin	76 ml	0.76 ml

Procedure

1. Melt the white paraffin and coconut oil.
2. Add liquid paraffin previously warmed at the same temperature and mix (A).
3. Disperse the coal tar in the polysorbate 80.
4. Incorporate the salicylic acid and mix with the previously melted emulsifying wax (B).
5. Add (A) with stirring to the (B) mix thoroughly and stir until cold.

Category: Local irritant.

Storage: Preserve in a well-closed container, protect from light.

Uses: Local irritant, disinfectant.

It is used for topical treatment of conditions like acne, seborrheic dermatitis, psoriasis, warts, corns, calluses and hyperkeratotic skin disorders.

EXPERIMENT 22

Object: To prepare and submit 5 boric acid suppositories.

Principle: Suppositories are conical or ovoid, solid preparations for insertion into the rectum where they melt dissolve or disperse and exert a local or less often, a systemic effect. Their basis is fat, a wax or a glycerol-gelatin jelly. They weigh 1, 2 or occasionally 4 g. Earlier, small suppositories known, as cones were prescribed for ear infections and long, very narrow forms, called bougies, were used for nasal and urethral infections.

There are virtually absolute today. Medicaments are prescribed in suppositories for these reasons:
1. To exert a direct action on the rectum.
2. To promote evacuation of the bowel.
3. To provide a systemic effect.

Systemic treatment by the rectal route is of particular value for:

   a. Treating patients who are unconscious, mentally disturbed or unable to tolerate oral medication because of vomiting or pathological conditions of the alimentary tract.
   b. Administering drugs, that cause gastric irritation, such as aminophylline.
   c. To produce mechanical action on the lower bowel and facilitate evacuation in the treatment of hemorrhoids, anal irritation, constipation, etc.
   d. Treating infants.

Suppositories are usually prepared by melting a suitable base, incorporating the prescribed amounts of finely powdered medicament(s) and pouring the mixture into moulds.

Displacement value: The volume of suppository that occupy in a given mould remains same. The weight of a medicated suppository varies when compared to a plain suppository. It is due to the variation of the densities of the medicament and the base. It means the weight of the medicament may not displace the same weight of the base for the same volume. Therefore, an allowance is made for the alteration in the density of the total mass, due to the added medicament. It is calculated by applying displacement value.

Calculation is done for extra quantity to manipulate the loss during preparation. Boric acid is insoluble in cocoa-butter. Therefore mixed with a portion of melted cocoa butter on a warm tile. The warm tile prevents the cooling and solidification of the base during mixing only 2/3 of the base is melted, as this prevents over heating of the base and the formation of unsatisfactory suppositories. When cocoa butter is heated above its melting temperature (about 36°C) and chilled to its solidification point (below 15°C), immediately after returning to room temperature this cocoa butter attains a melting point of about 24°C, therefore cocoa butter must not be heated at higher temperature. Cooling the mould dissipates the contain heat and hastens settling of the base. Over filling of the mould is done to prevent hollows and depressions forming at top of the suppository due to contraction of the base.

Observation Table

S. No	Ingredients	Quantity given	Quantity taken
1.	Boric acid	120 mg	600 mg
2.	Cocoa-butter q.s	1 g	5 g

Note: Displacement value of boric acid is 1.5

Procedure: Clean the suppository mould with hot water and detergent. Lubricate the mould with the lubricant fluid and invert the mould in ice. Weigh the cocoa butter and transfer to a china dish. Melt 2/3 of it on a water bath, remove from the water bath and stir well with until all that has melted.

Warm a small tile on a water bath. Place the boric acid on the warmed tile. Pour half of the melted base on the boric acid powder on the tile and mix well to get a smooth dispersion. Transfer the dispersion to the porcelain dish and stir well to form a homogeneous mixture.

Fill 6 cavities of the mould to overflow. Allow the mass to set. Trim of the excess with a sharp blade. Keep the mould for half an hour on ice. Open the mould and remove the suppositories. Blot off the excess lubricant.

Select the 5 best suppositories wrap and dispense in a neatly labelled box.

Category: Local anti-infective.

Storage: Store in a cool place.

Direction: For rectal use only.

Uses: As an antifungal and antibacterial.

EXPERIMENT 23

Object: To prepare and submit 5 zinc oxide suppositories.

Principle: Same as of boric acid suppositories.

Observation Table

S. No	Ingredients	Quantity given	Quantity taken
1.	Zinc oxide	600 mg	3 g
2.	Cocoa-butter q.s	2 g	10 g

Note: Displacement value of zinc oxide is 5.

Procedure

1. Calculate the quantities required, taking displacement values into account if relevant. Excess must be made because of unavoidable wastage during preparation.
2. Select a dry, clean mould and place it on a clean tile.
3. Shred the fat with a fine food grater. Weigh the required amount, avoiding lumps that will be slow to melt, and place in the smelliest evaporating basin that will hold it. The shreds can be poled high because the volume contracts considerably on melting. A porcelain dish is preferable because it is easier to overheat the contents in a metal type
4. Finely powder the medicaments and pass each through a separate number 180 sieve. Weigh the required quantities.
5. Heat a small tile until it is comfortably warm to the hand. If this is done over a water bath, dry the tile thoroughly afterwards.
6. Mix the powders on the tile with a flexible spatula.
7. Place the base on the water bath until about two-thirds of the contents has melted and then remove from the heat the rest will melt with stirring, particularly if the dish is tightly cupped in the palm of one hand. Stir with a small, non-tapering spatula; not a glass rod, because base tends to solidify on the stirrer and is more easily removed from a spatula onto the edge of the dish. Overheating may occur if the base is left over the heat until completely melted.
8. Pour about half of the melted base onto the mixed medicaments and work into a smooth dispersion as quickly as possible by levigating with the spatula. Avoid loss over the edge of the tile. To prevent excessive cooling through spreading over a large area, use as small a tile as is consistent with avoidance of spillage. If the base solidifies it can be softened by holding the tile over the water bath for a few seconds.

9. Transfer the disoperation to the dish, leaving virtually none on the tile, and air to form a homogeneous mixture.

10. Continue stirring until the mixture begins to thicken. Then fill each cavity of the mould to overflowing. Meanwhile stir the mass continuously; this precaution (easily forgotten due to anxiety that setting will take place before the mould is filled), and delay in pouring until the mass is about to sedimentation of insoluble solids. If necessary, use the spatula to help the viscous base from the dish. Should solidification occur during pouring, apply the minimum of heat to start the mass moving again. The cavities are overfilled to prevent depressions in the tops of the suppositories due to contraction of the base during cooling.

11. Leave for two or three minutes until the mass has just not and then remove the excess from the mould with a sharp knife, razor blade or a slightly warm spatula.

12. Leave in a cool place for 10 to 15 minutes. Then open the mould and remove the suppositories. If any are difficult to separate, reclose the mould loosely and tap the base squarely and firmly on the protected bench, a procedure that generally force suppositories of the synthetic for type.

Note

- The large amount of powder in this preparation cannot be incorporated satisfactorily in a 1 g suppository; hence, the official product is made in a 2 g mould.
- Preferably, these suppositories should be made with a synthetics fatty base but it is interesting to prepare them with theobroma oil for experience in the problems presented with this base.
- To obtain a homogeneous suppository of uniform composition and colour it is advisable to levigate the powders with a little water before mixing with the base. About 0.4 ml per suppository is suitable but this must be taken into account when calculating the amount of base required.

Category: Local anti-infective.

Storage: Store in a cool place.

Direction: For rectal use only.

Uses: As an antifungal and antibacterial.

EXPERIMENT 24

Object: To prepare and submit 100 ml of paracetamol pediatric elixir IP.

Principle: Elixirs are clear, flavoured hydroalcoholic preparation intended for oral use. They contain one or more medicament, pleasantly flavoured usually attractively coloured containing high proportion of alcohol or sucrose along with some suitable antimicrobial agent. The alcoholic content in elixir vary from 5–40%. In general they are more stable than mixture as sufficient alcohol is added to maintain the drug in the solution.

Elixirs are of Two Types

1. **Non-medicated elixirs:** They are used purely as diluting agents or solvents for drugs containing approximately 25% alcohol, e.g. simple elixirs is alcoholic elixirs or low alcohol elixirs (containing 7–10% alcohol), high alcoholic elixirs (containing 60–75% alcohol).

2. **Medicated elixirs:** Elixirs containing therapeutically active compounds are known as medicated elixirs, e.g. phenobarbital elixirs USP, dexamethasone elixirs USP chloropheniramine maleate elixirs.

Observation Table

S. No	Ingredients	Quantity given	Quantity taken
1.	Paracetamol	24 ml	2.4 ml
2.	Ethanol (96%)	100 ml	10 ml
3.	Propylene glycol	100 ml	10 ml
4.	Concentrated raspberry juice	25 ml	2 ml
5.	Chloroform spirit	20 ml	2 ml
6.	Invert sugar	275 ml	27.5 ml
7.	Amaranth solutio	2 ml	0.2 ml
8.	Glycerine	1000 ml (qs)	100 ml (qs)

Procedure

1. Mix ethanol (96%), propylene glycol and choloroform spirit and make a mixture.

2. Dissolve paracetamol and shake it, add other additives.

3. Finally and sufficient amount of glycerin to produce 1000 ml.

Category: Antipyretic.

Storage: Preserve in a well-closed container, protect from light.

Uses: Analgesic and antipyretic, used to bring down the elevated temperature.

EXPERIMENT 25

Object: To prepare 100g of ORS powder (IP), label it and dispense it in a suitable container.

Theory: A pharmaceutical powder is a mixture of finely divided drug and or chemicals in dry form. These are solid dosage form of medicament, which are meant for internal and external use. They are available in crystalline or amorphous form. The particle size of powder plays an important role in physical, chemical and biological properties of the dosage forms. There is a relationship between particle size of powder and dissolution, absorption and therapeutic efficacy of drugs.

Powders are classified as:

1. Bulk powder for external use
2. Bulk powders for internal use
3. Simple and compound powders
4. Effervescent granules
5. Cachets.

Materials: Beaker, weight box, mortar and pestle, sieve number 80.

Reagents: sodium chloride, potassium chloride, sodium bicarbonate, dextrose.

Formula

S. No	Ingredients	Quantity given	Quantity taken
1.	Sodium chloride	12.5 g	3.5 g
2.	Potassium chloride	5.35 g	1.49 g
3.	Sodium bicarbonate	10.3 g	2.88 g
4.	Dextrose	71.4 g	19.9 g

Calculation

1. 100 g powder contains 12.5 g of sodium chloride

$$28 \text{ g powder contains} = \frac{12.5 \times 28}{100} = 3.5 \text{ g}$$

2. 100 g powder contains 5.35 g of potassium chloride

$$28 \text{ g powder contains} = \frac{5.35 \times 28}{100} = 1.49 \text{ g}$$

3. 100 g powder contains 10.3 g of. sodium bicarbonate

$$28 \text{ g powder contains} = \frac{10.3 \times 28}{100} = 2.88 \text{ g}$$

4. 100 g powder contains 71.4 g of dextrose

$$28 \text{ g powder contains} = \frac{71.4 \times 28}{100} = 19.9 \text{ g}$$

Procedure

1. Weigh the required amount of sodium chloride, potassium chloride, sodium bicarbonate, and dextrose.
2. Mix them in mortar and pestle and pass through the sieve number 80.
3. Dispense the powder and label it.

   Category: As a electrolytic.

   Storage: Stored in a well-closed airtight container keep it in a cool and dry place.

Uses

1. Used in dehydration, dysentery and diarrhea.
2. As a electrolyte replenisher.

EXPERIMENT 26

Object: To prepare 100 g of absorbable dusting powder (USP/NF), label it and dispense it in a suitable container.

Theory: Dusting powder is powder in a fine state of subdivision of such substance for external application. They are usually mixture of substance zinc oxide, starch and boric acid or natural mineral substance such as kaolin or talc the later may be contaminated with pathogenic organism and should therefore be sterilized by heat. Dusting powders are not intended for oral use. Dusting powder should be passed through sieve number 80 (#80) before dusting to avoid partial loss. It is better to weigh for some extra quantity, dusting powders are two types.

1. Medical
2. Surgical

Materials: Beaker and, weight box, mortar and pestle, sieve number 80

Reagents: Zinc oxide, starch, salicylic acid, talc.

Formula

S. No	Ingredients	Quantity given	Quantity taken
1.	Purified talc	500 g	50 g
2.	Starch	250 g	25 g
3.	Zinc oxide	50 g	5 g
4.	Salicylic acid	200 g	20 g

Calculation

1. 1000 g powder contain 500 g of purified talc.

Hence 100 g powder contains $= \dfrac{500 \times 100}{1000} = 50\,g$

2. 1000 g powder contain 250 g of starch.

Hence 100 g powder contain $= \dfrac{250 \times 100}{1000} = 25\,g$

3. 1000 g powder contain 50 g of zinc oxide.

Hence 100 g powder contains $= \dfrac{50 \times 100}{1000} = 5\,g$

4. 1000 g powder contain 200 g of salicylic acid.

Hence 100 g powder contains $= \dfrac{200 \times 100}{1000} = 20\,g$

Procedure

1. Weigh the required quantity of starch, talc, zinc oxide and salicylic acid.

2. Mix them in ascending order of their weight.
3. Pass the mix powder through a sieve number 80.
4. After sieving, again mix the contents.
5. Dispense dusting powder in six sub-divided glass, label and dispense it.

Category: As medical and surgical.

Storage: "Store in a cool and dry place".

Uses

1. As an antiperspirant.

Glossary

Absorption: The assimilation of one substance by another, where the substance being absorbed diffuses into the absorbing material.

Acid: A chemical compound containing a hydrogen atom that dissociates from a molecule to a hydronium ion in water.

Adsorption: The attachment of one substance onto the surface of another by means of a strong interaction between the two substances or materials. This differs from absorption in that the substances are joined only at the surface.

Aerosol: A dispersion of very small (submicron) sized liquid droplets or solid particles into a gas. The term is used in packaging as a label for all liquid or semisolid solutions or suspensions dispensed under pressure.

Amorphous: Not crystalline when used with plastics, it means molecules arranged in a random order, without structure.

Ampoule: Glass tubing sealed at both ends, containing a drug intended for injection.

Analgesic: A substance that relieves pain.

ANDA: Abbreviated New Drug Application.

Anesthetic: A drug that stops or suppresses sensations, such as pain by affecting either the central nervous system (general anesthetic) or the peripheral nerve structures (local anesthetic).

Angina: A heart disease characterized by intermittent chest pain coupled with feelings of suffocation.

Angstrom: A unit of length equal to one hundred millionth of a centimeter.

Annealing: A controlled temperature method of gradually cooling glass containers in ovens to relieve structural stresses and to make the glass less brittle.

Antibiotics: Substances that inhibit the growth of or destroy microorganisms.

Antihistamines: Substances that neutralize or inhibit the effects of histamine released by the body during allergic reactions or in response to a disease.

Anti-inflammatory: Substances that neutralize or inhibit the inflammation of tissue.

Antimicrobial: Refers to substances that destroy microorganisms.

Antioxidant: A chemical substance that can be added to a plastic resin to minimize or prevent the effects of oxygen attack on the plastic (e.g. yellowing or degradation).

Antipruritic: A substance that relieves itching.

Antiseptic: A substance that inhibits the growth of microorganisms.

Antistatic agent: A chemical substance that can be applied to the surface of a plastic bottle or incorporated in the plastic from which the bottle is made. Its function is to render the surface of the plastic article less susceptible to an accumulation of electrostatic charges, which attract and hold fine dust on the surface of the bottle.

API: Active pharmaceutical ingredient—the active ingredient in a pharmaceutical product.

Aseptic: Free from disease-producing microorganisms. In biologic or medical applications, it refers to an operation performed in a presterilized environment that is controlled to prevent contamination through the introduction of microorganisms. Sterile area that is controlled to remain sterile during operation.

Aseptic filling: The process of combining sterilized pharmaceuticals with sterile packaged in a sterile environment.

Assay: The determination of the concentration of the active ingredient in a pharmaceutical.

Astringent: A substance that contracts tissues or canals, reducing the discharge of fluids.

Autoclave: A vessel capable of containing high-pressure steam that is commonly used to sterilize pharmaceuticals, medical instruments, and medical devices.

Bactericide: A substance that kills bacteria.

Bacteriostat: A substance that is added to a drug formulation to control the growth of bacteria.

Base: A chemical compound that when dissolved in water dissociates to form a hydroxyl ion and raises pH above 7. Generally a metal oxide or hydroxide.

Bioavailability: The availability of an administered drug to the circulatory system.

Blank: The mold parts used in all glass container machines for preliminary formation of glass in preparation for completion of the glass containers in the finish mold where the bottles are blown. The blank forms the parison; hence, the parison itself is at times referred to as the blank.

Blister package: A package consisting of a cavity thermoformed from a thermoplastic material and a flat lid stock designed to seal each of the cavities to the edges of the trimmed card.

BTU: British thermal unit.

Buccal cavity: The cavity formed by the cheek.

Buffer: A buffer is a substance that when dissolved in water acts to resist changed in pH that would otherwise be caused by environmental factors (e.g. CO_2 in air or alkaline salts in glass containers).

CAD/CAM: Computer-assisted design/computer-assisted manufacturing (or in printing computer-assisted makeup).

Caplet: A tablet-shaped capsule.

Capsule: A transparent or coloured gelatin material, hard- or soft-shelled that contains a drug preparation.

Catalyst: A chemical compound that accelerates the rate of a chemical reaction without being consumed in the process.

CGMP: Current Good Manufacturing Practice (as written and used outside the FDA).

Coefficient of thermal expansion: A dimensionless number that expresses the degree to which a material will expand when subjected to a known and specified increase in temperature.

Copolymer: A polymer made from at least two different comonomers.

Cosmetic: Formulate products used to decorate, adorn, or beautify but which have no therapeutic effect or purpose.

Cream: A medicated preparation based on an emulsion of oil in water.

Deliquescence: Refers to a substance that readily absorbs moisture. Becoming damp or liquid by absorption of water from the atmosphere and then dissolving in the water taken up. This property is found in salts (e.g. $CaCl_2$).

Demulcent: A substance formulated to soothe the part of the body to which it is applied.

Densitometer: For printing, a reflection densitometer is used to measure and control the density of colour inks on a substrate.

Density: Weight per unit of volume of a substance.

Depyrogenation: The elimination of pyrogens by heat or chemical processes.

Dermatological: Pertaining to the skin or diseases of the skin.

Die: Any tool or arrangement of tools designed to cut, shape, or otherwise form materials to a desired configuration.

Distillation: The process in which a liquid is purified by transforming it into a vapor, separating the vapor from the impure liquid and then condensing and collecting it.

Diuretic: A drug formulation that increases urinary discharge.

DMF: Drug Master File, a blinded repository for proprietary information that permits the FDA to review the safety and adequacy of a component.

Dosage form: The form of a drug preparation that determines how the drug is administered (e.g. tablet, oral liquid, suppository, parenteral liquid).

Effervescent: Refers to substances that produce a gas, usually CO_2, upon mixing with water.

Efflorescent: Refers to substances that lose water on exposure to air.

EFPIA: European Federation of Pharmaceutical Industries and Associations.

EHIBCC: Health Industry Business Communication Council (HIBCC) and its affiliate International Organization, the European Health Industry Business Communications Council.

Elastomer: A polymer with the elastic characteristics similar to rubber: the ability to best retched to at least twice its original length without sustaining permanent deformation.

Elixirs: Syrups containing 20 to 25% alcohol.

EMEA: The European Agency for the Evaluation of Medicinal Products.

Emollients: Substances that soften and relax the tissues when applied locally.

Emulsion: A liquid consisting of a discontinuous, immiscible liquid phase dispersed in a continuous liquid phase.

Enteric: Refers to coatings that delay dissolution until a solid dosage form reaches the intestine.

FD and C: Food, Drug, and Cosmetic Act.

FDA: United States Food and Drug Administration.

FFDCA: Federal Food, Drug, and Cosmetic Act.

Filtration: The process by which solid particles are removed from a liquid by passing the liquid through a porous medium whose pores are so small that the solid particles will not pass through them.

Flint: A term used to describe a glass color that is perfectly clear and transparent.

Fluidized bed: A group of solid particles in a container that are agitated by the upward flowing stream of gas. The particles appear as a cloud in the bottom of the confining space.

Fluorocarbon: An organic compound containing fluorine.

Flux: A substance or mixture used to promote the fusion of metals or minerals. Can be called a fluxing agent.

Free radical: A highly reactive species formed by the rupture of a chemical bond.

Gastrointestinal: The system of body organs that included the stomach and small intestine.

Gel: A colloidal semisolid consisting of a networked structure of suspended, fine, solid particles surrounded by a liquid. Differs from a colloidal solution, which has no solid particles to confer some rigidity to the structure.

Gelatin: A water soluble substance extracted from animal tissue and bones and used in the manufacturing of capsules.

Generic: Used in the pharmaceutical business to describe any drug that is labelled for sale with its technical name rather than a trade name, and usually manufactured by companies that were not the original developer of the product.

Glass: The USP on the basis of performance in chemical durability tests specifies four types of glass. Type 1, 2, and 3 are intended for packaging parenteral preparations and type NP for nonparenteral products.

HDPE: High-density polyethylene.

Head space: The space between the level of the contents of a container and the closure of the container.

Hermetic seal: Any seal or any container so sealed that is impervious to all gasses under normal conditions of handling and storage.

HIBCC: Health Industry Business Communication Council and its affiliate international organization, the European Health Industry Business Communications Council (EHIBCC).

Hologram: The image formed by a lensless photographic process (holography) that uses laser light to produce three-dimensional images.

Hormone: A substance formed in and secreted by the endocrine glands. May be made synthetically.

Hydrocarbon: An organic compound containing only carbon and hydrogen.

Hydrolysis: Reaction of a compound with water, resulting in destruction of the compound and the formation of at least two new ones.

Hypertonic: Having a greater osmotic pressure than blood plasma, lacrimal fluid, or interstitial fluid. It can be applied more specifically to a fluid in which cells shrink.

Hypoglycemia: An abnormally small concentration of glucose in the circulating blood.

In vitro: Refers to chemical or physical tests of drugs using laboratory procedures and apparatus (in glass).

In vivo: Refers to tests of drugs in laboratory tissue, animals, and humans (in life).

IND: Investigational New Drug.

Induction heating: Heating a metal object by application of an external magnetic field to generate heat-producing eddy currents in the object.

Infusion: Introduction of a fluid other than blood into a vein (e.g. a saline solution drip).

Inhalant: A substance that can be vaporized by mechanical means or by heat and carried into the respiratory tract by inhalation.

Intravenous: Administration of a drug by injection directly into a vein.

Ion: A charged atom or group of atoms formed by the dissociation of a molecule, often in an aqueous medium.

IQ: Installation qualification. This is a review of the equipment that establishes that the equipment meets its design specifications, and was installed in accordance with the design specifications. A term used in validation.

IR: Infrared.

Isotonic: Solutions that have the same osmotic pressure. A more specific definition is a solution in which cells neither swell nor shrink.

Isotonicity: The situation obtained when the colligative or osmotic properties of a pharmaceutical are matched with those of a biological site of administration, frequently mucous membranes.

IV: Intravenous.

Kaolin: A family of clays containing combinations of hydrated alumina and silica.

Keratolytic: A medication used to treat conditions that lead to horny skin growths.

Kpsi: 1000 psi.

Latex: The milky juice of exudation of plants obtained by tapping the trunk (e.g. the fluid from a rubber plant).

LDPE: Low-density polyethylene.

Light-resistant container: A container that protects the contents from the effects of light.

Lipophilic: Having a strong affinity for oily or fatty substances.

LLDPE: Linear low-density polyethylene.

Lot or lot number: A lot refers to all the products made during a single run or manufacturing sequence on a piece of equipment or a complete production line. A run may last for a given quantity, for hours, or days, it normally denotes all products made in one sequence of starting and stopping the equipment when all raw materials are consumed or a given quantity is produced. A lot number is the assigned designation of that specific manufacturing sequence.

Lyophilization: Freeze-drying. The removal of water or solvent from a substance by applying a vacuum to the substance after it has been frozen.

Magma: Highly thickened suspensions for oral administration.

Mandrel: A metal rod or bar used as a core around which metal, glass, etc. is cast molded or shaped.

mg: Milligram.

Microbial control: Assembly of products in a controlled clean environment, followed by exposure to gamma radiation. This process reduces bioburden load but does not support a "sterile" label claim.

Microencapsulation: The encasement of small particles, either solid or liquid, within a shell that prevents their escape until the shell is ruptured by an external force or dissolved by a solvent.

Micron: One ten-thousandth of a centimeter.

Microorganisms, microbes: Living microscopic entities including bacteria and molds.

Multiple-dose container: A multiple-unit container for parenteral or ophthalmic formulations.

Multiple-unit container: One that permits the withdrawal of part of the contents while containing and protecting the un-withdrawn balance.

NDA: New Drug Application (FDA). Submission of all information necessary for review by the agency prior to approval of a new drug.

NDC: National Drug Code.

NF: National Formulary.

NWDA: The National Wholesale Druggists Association.

OFAS: Office of Food Additive Safety.

Offset: The process of using an intermediate cylinder to transfer an image from the image center to the substrate.

Ointment: A medicated preparation with the oleaginous base. More generally, a semisolid preparation intended for topical administration.

Oleaginous base: A base with the nature or quality of an oil.

ONPLDS: Office of Nutritional Products, Labeling, and Dietary Supplements.

Ophthalmic: Related to the eye.

OPP: Oriented polypropylene.

OTC: Over the counter.

Otic: Related to the ear.

Oxidation: Reaction with oxygen, more generally removal of electrons from an atom or molecule.

Parenteral: Introduction of substances into an organism by subcutaneous, intramuscular, intravenous, or intramedullary injection. Introduction by some other means than through the gastrointestinal tract.

pH: A measure of the hydrogen ion concentration in and the acidity of an aqueous solution.

Pharmaceutical: A manufactured, processed, or compounded form of a drug.

PIM: Product information management.

Plasticizer: A substance mixed into a plastic to decrease its stiffness and increase its softness.

Polymer: A high molecular weight molecule formed by reacting small molecules (monomers) together to form a long chain consisting of many monomer units.

Polyolefin: Any polymer whose monomer units are unsaturated hydrocarbons (olefins) containing only carbon and hydrogen. Polyethylene and polypropylene are the most common polyolefins used in packaging.

PPB: Parts per billion.

Prophylaxis: Prevention of disease or its spread by the administration of drugs and/or procedures.

Protocol: A set of procedures. Test or validation protocols are the set of instructions that govern how a test is run and how the data is to be reported.

PTFE: Polytetrafluoroethylene.

PVC: Polyvinyl chloride.

PVDC: Polyvinylidene chloride.

Pyrogen: Agent that causes a rise in body temperature, especially if injected. The most important pyrogen in sterile drug manufacture is endotoxins, a residue from gram-negative bacteria.

Resin: The term for a polymer in the form of small pellets that is packaged in a bag or in bulk and shipped to a processor. Sometimes a direct reference to the polymer itself.

Reverse osmosis: The process in which the solute in a solution is removed by forcing the solvent, against the normal osmotic pressure to flow through a membrane that is not permeable to the solute. Used to remove salts from seawater.

RH: Relative humidity.

Saturated: When used to describe a type of chemical bond or molecule, the bonding is saturated if no double or triple bonds exist, i.e. each atom is joined within the molecule to other atoms only by single bonds.

Scabacide: A substance that destroys the organism causing scabies.

Secondary package: The package that contains the primary package. It is not in direct contact with the product. Usually a box or carton.

Semipermeable-membrane: A membrane that permits the passage of one or more components of a solution but does not allow the passage of other components. Such membranes are usually permeable only by the solvent.

Shelf-life: The time required for the potency of a drug to drop to 90% of its labelled potency.

Single-dose container: A single-unit container for primarily used for parenterals but also for other dosage forms that contains only one dose of product.

Single-unit container: A container that holds the quantity of drug intended for administration as a single dose promptly after the container is opened.

Sol: A colloidal solution or liquid phase of a colloidal solution.

Sterile: The absence of microorganisms.

Sterility testing: Tests performed to determine whether viable microorganisms are present. Commonly, the test involves immersing a component or system or flushing a fluid pathway with sterile microbial growth medium, incubation of the medium under conditions favourable for microbial growth, and observation of turbidity or other indication of microbial growth after a suitable incubation period.

Sterilization: A validated process used to render a product free from viable microorganisms. It is generally accepted that a terminally sterilized unit purporting to be sterile attain a sterility assurance level of 10–6, i.e. probability of less than or equal to one chance in 1 million that a viable microorganism is present in the sterilized unit. Lower SALs may be validated as sterile in some cases.

Steroid: Fat-soluble organic compounds, such as sterols, bile acids, and sex hormones.

Stratum corneum: The outermost layer of skin.

Strip package: A package made by enclosing an object to be packaged, such as a tablet between two webs and then sealing the webs together so that the seal completely surrounds the object being packaged.

Subcutaneous: Beneath the skin.

Sublingual: Under the tongue.

Substrate: Refers to the primary structural material or the surface of the primary material that is applied to other materials designed to alter the characteristics or properties of the original material.

Suppository: The dosage form designed for insertion into the rectum.

Surfactant: Any substance, normally a soap or detergent, that forms a compatibilizing boundary layer between two liquids or a liquid and solid. This layer leads to the staple dispersion one phase in another.

Suspension: Solid particles dispersed in a liquid. If the suspension is stable, it will resist the normal gravitational separation into two phases.

Systemic: Administration of a drug so that it gains access to the circulatory system. Can also refer to the introduction of a drug to all parts of the body to treat only one location.

Tensile strength: The resistance of a specimen to breaking when stressed longitudinally.

Therapeutic: Relating to the treatment of disease.

Thermoplastic: Describes any substance that becomes more pliable as it is heated. In packaging and molding, it refers to a material that can be formed when hot but become rigid after cooling.

Thermoset: Plastics that become rigid when heated or subjected to energy that initiates a chemical reaction at reactive sites linking all the individual polymer strands together permanently.

Tight container: A term defined by the USP that describes a container that protects its contents from contamination by extraneous liquids, solids, or gases from physical loss of the drug and from efflorescence, deliquescence, or evaporating under ordinary or customary conditions of handling, shipment, storage, and distribution.

Tincture: A solution of a drug in alcohol.

Topical: Administration of a drug to the skin surface or the lining of body cavities. Its effectiveness is limited to the localized areas to which it is applied.

Toxin: A noxious or poisonous substance formed during the growth of certain microorganisms.

Toxoid: A toxin that has been treated, e.g. with formaldehyde to destroy its toxic property but retain its antigenicity, i.e. its capability of stimulating the production of antitoxin antibodies and thus engendering immunity.

Transdermal: Administration of drugs through the skin.

Type I glass: Glass composed largely of silica and boric oxide that is very low in water extractable impurities.

Type II glass: Glass containing larger amounts of water-soluble sodium and calcium oxides than type I glass. Soda-lime glass with no boron-containing materials present.

Type III glass: Glass containing even greater quantities of water-extractable oxides than type II glass. A different and lower grade of soda-lime glass.

Unit-dose container: A single-unit container for products for administration by other than parenteral means as a singe dose direct from the container.

Unsaturated: In chemistry, molecules that contain more than one bond between two atoms. In polymers, it is usually referring to double and triple bonds between carbon and another atom.

USP: United States Pharmacopoeia.

USP-NF: United States Pharmacopoeia National Formulary.

UV: Ultraviolet.

Validation: Testing and establishing documented evidence that provides a high degree of assurance that a specific process, component, or piece of equipment will consistently produce a product meeting its predetermined specifications and quality attributes.

Vasoconstrictors: Drugs that reduce the flow of body fluids by constricting the ducts, tubes, and canals through which these fluids flow. Often referred to drugs that constrict the circulatory system.

Vasodilators: Drugs that increase the flow of body fluids by relaxing the muscles surrounding the ducts, tubes, and canals through which those fluids flow.

Wavelength: The distance between identical points in a wave pattern. A measure of the energy content of light, the shorter the wavelength the higher the energy level.

Well-closed container: A USP term. A container that protects its contents from extraneous solids and physical loss under the ordinary and customary conditions of handling, shipment, and distribution.

Appendices

APPENDIX 1

List of some commonly used additives

ABSORBENTS

Bentonite	Magnesium silicate
Kaolin	Silica (cab-o-sil, syloid, aerosil)
Magnesium carbonate	Starch
Magnesium oxide	Tricalcium phosphate

ANTIADHESIVES

Colloidal silica	Metallic stearates
Corn starch	Sodium lauryl sulfate
DL-Leucine	Talc
Magnesium stearate	

ANTIFOAMING AGENTS

Ariacel C	GMS
Atlas G 1706	Propylene glycol monostearate
Ethylene glycol fatty acid ester	Span 65
(Emcol EC-50)	Span 85

ANTIOXIDANTS

Acetone	Maleic Acid
Ascorbic acid	Monoisopropylcitrate
Ascorbyl palmitate	Nor-dihydroguaiaretic acid
Benzoin	Phenyl alphanapthlamine
Beta-naphthol	Propyl gallate
Butylated hydroxytoluene	Pyrogallol
Butylated hydroxyanisole	Pyrocatechol
Citric acid	Sodium bisulfite
Cysteine hydrochloride	Sodium formaldehyde sulfoxylate

Dilauryl thiodipropionate

Distearylthiodipropionate

Ethylgallate

Gallic acid

Glycerin

Guaiac resin

Hydroquinon

Isoascorbic acid

Lecithin

Sodium metabisulfite

Sodium sulfite

Sodium thiosulfate

Thioglycerol

Thiosolbitol

Thiourea

Thioglycollic acid

Alpha tocopherol

Trihydroxybutyrophenone

COLOURS

1. Natural

Alizarin

Anattenes

Caramel

Beta-carotene

Carbon black

Carmic acid

Chlorophyll

Cochineal

Curcumin

Ferric oxides (red and yellow)

Hesperidin

Indigo

Quercetin

Riboflavin

Rubia tinctorum

Rutin

Saffron

Titanium dioxide

Turmeric

Tyrian purple

2. Synthetic

Alizarin cyanine

Amaranth I N 16785

Brilliant Blue FCS 42090

Carmoisine 14720

Eosine G 45380

Erythorosin 45430

Fast red E 16045

Fast green FCF 42053

Green S 44090

Freen F 61570

Indigo carmine 73015

Napthol blue black 20470

Orange G 16 30

Ponceaux 4 16255

Quinazarine 61565

Quinoline yellow SS 47000

Resoroin brown 20170

Sudan III 26100

Sunset yello FCF 15185

Tartrazine 19140

EMULSIFYING AGENTS

1. Surfactants forming monomolecular films

Alkylpolyoxyethylene sulfates   Polyoxyethylene monolaurate
(Atlas G 2127)

Benzalkonium chloride	(Polyoxyethylene alkylphenol (lgepal CA 630)
Cetrimide	Polyoxyethylene sorbitan monolaurate (Tween 20)
Dioctylsodium sulfosuccinate	Polyoxyethylene sorbitan monopalmitate (Tween 40)
Lauryldimethylbenzylam-monium chloride	Polyoxyethylene sorbitan (Tween 80)
Lecithin	Polyoxyethylene laurylether (Brij 35)
N-cetyl N-ethyl morpholinium ethosulfate (Atlas G-263)	Monostearate (Myrj 52)
PEG 400 monostearate	Castor oil (Atlas G 1974)
Polyoxyethylene laurylether (Brij 30)	Potassium oleate
Polyoxyethylene monostearate (Myrj 45)	Sodium oleate
Propylene glycol monostearate	Sodium lauryl sulfate
Propylene glycol monostearate (Atlas G 917)	Sorbitan monopalmitate (Span 40)
Sorbitan monolaurate (Span 20)	Sorbitan monostearate (Arlacel 60)
Glyceryl monostearate (GMS)	Sodium laurate
Sorbitan sesquioleate (Alacel C)	Triethanolmine oleate
Potassium stearate	Triethanolamine stearate

2. **Surfactants forming multimolecular films**

Acacia	Hectorite
Agar	Magnesium hydroxide
Alginates	Pectin
Atapulgite	Silica gel
Bentonite	Tragacanth
Gelatin	Veegum

FLAVOURING AGENTS

Almond	Oil of anise
Amyl acetate	Oil of bergamot
Anethol	Oil of caraway
Apricot	Oil of cardamom
Apple	Oil of cinnamon

Banana	Oil of clove
Benzaldelyde	Oil of coriander
Black current	Oil of fennel
Blueberry	Oil of lemon
Butterscotch	Oil of lavender
Burgundy	Oil of nutmeg
Cherry	Oil of orange
Chocolate	Oil of narcissus
Custard	Oil of peppermint
Ethyl acetate	Oil of rosemary
Ethyl vanillin	Oil of rose
Eucalyptol	Oil of spearmint
Eugenol	Oil of thyme
Ginger	Orris root
Hyacinth	Peach
Jasmine	Pheyl ethyl alcohol
Lemongrass	Pineapple
Liquorice	Plum
Mango	Raspberry
Maple	Samdalwood
Methyl salicylate	Saffron
Melon	Strawberry
Narcissus	Thymol
Neroli	Vanillin
Violet	

FLOCCULATING AGENTS

Electrolytes like KH_2PO_4 $AlCl_3$ NaCl, etc.	Ionic and non ionic surfactants Hydrocolloids

PRESERVATIVES

Banzalkonium chloride	Boric acid and propyl alcohol
Benzoic acid and benzoates	Cetrimide
Benzylalcohol	Dichlorophene
Cetylpyridinium chloride	Ortho and parachlorbenzoic acid
Chlorbutanol	Parahydroxybenzoates
Chlorothymol	Parachlor metacresol
p-Chlorphenylglyceryl ether	Parachlor metaxylenol
Dichlorometasylenol	p-Chlor phenylpropanediol
Dehydroacetic acid of phyenylmercuric acid	Phenyl mercuric nitrate and other salts

Formic acid	Phenol
Formaldehyde	Phenol hexachlorophene

SOLUBILISING AGENTS

Atlas G 1690	PEG 400 monostearate
Atlas G 1794	Sodium oleate
Brij 35	Triethanolamine oleate
Igepal CA 630	Tween 20
Myrj 45	Tween 40
Myrj 49	Tween 60
Myrj 51	Tween 80
Myrj 52	

SUSPENDING AGENTS

Acacia	Hectorite
Agar	Hydroxyethyl cellulose
Alginates	Hydroxyl propyl cellulose
Attapulgite	Methyl celluloses
Bentonite	Microcrystalline cellulose
Carboxy methyl celluloses	Polyvinyl alcohol
Carbopol	Povidone
Carbomer	Psyllium seed gum
Cellulose poweder	Pectin
Chondorus	Tragacanth
Gelatin	Veegum
Guar gum	

SWEETENING AGENTS

Aspartyl phenylalanie	Maltose
Cyclamates	Mannitol
Dextrose	Neohsperidin dehydrochalone
Fructose	Saccharin
Glycerin	Sorbitol
Glycyrrhizin	Sucrose
Honey	Xylitol
Lactose	

WETTING AGENTS

Tween 20	Span 20
Brij 30	Span 40

APPENDIX 2
Units and conversion factors

Length	1 inch	$= 0.0254$ m
	1 ft	$= 0.3048$ m
Area	1 ft^2	$= 0.0929$ m^2
Volume	1 ft^3	$= 0.0283$ m^3
	1 gal Imp	$= 0.004546$ m^3
	1 gal US	$= 0.003785$ m^3 = 3.785 litres
	1 litre	$= 0.001$ m^3
Mass	1 lb	$= 0.4536$ kg
	1 mole	Molecular weight in kg
Density	1 lb/ft^3	$= 16.03$ kg m^{-3}
Velocity	1 ft/sec	$= 0.3048$ m s^{-1}
Pressure	1 lb/m^2	$= 6894$ Pa
	1 torr	$= 133.3$ Pa
	1 atm	$= 1.013 \times 10^5$ Pa = 760 mm Hg
	1 Pa	$= 1$ N m^{-2} = 1 kg m^{-1} s^{-2}
Force	1 Newton 1 lb ft s^{-2}	$= 1$ kg m s^{-2} = 1.49 kg m s^{-2}
Viscosity	1 cP	$= 0.001$ N s m^{-2} = 0.001 Pa s
	1 lb/ft sec	$= 1.49$ N s m^{-2} = 1.49 kg m^{-1} s^{-2}
Energy	1 Btu	$= 1055$ J
	1 cal	$= 4.186$ J
Power	1 kW 1 W	$= 1$ kJ s^{-1} = 1 J s^{-1}
	1 horsepower	$= 745.7$ W = 745.7 J s^{-1} = 0.746 kW
	1 ton refrigeration	$= 3.519$ kW
Temperature units	(°F)	$= 5/9$ (°C) = 5/9 (K)
Heat-transfer coefficient	1 Btu ft^{-2} h^{-1}°F^{-1}	$= 5.678$ J m^{-2} s^{-1}°C
Thermal conductivity	1 Btu ft^{-1} h^{-1}°F^{-1}	$= 1.731$ J m^{-1} s^{-1}°C^{-1}
Constants	Π	3.1416
	e (base of natural logs)	2.7183
	R	8.314 kJ mole^{-1} K^{-1} or 0.08206 m^3 atm mole^{-1} K^{-1}

(M) Mega $= 10^6$, (k) kilo $= 10^3$, (H) Hecto $= 10^2$, (m) milli $= 10^{-3}$, (μ) micro $= 10^{-6}$

APPENDIX 3

Standard sieves

S. No	Aperture $(m \times 10^{-3})$	ISO nominal aperture $(m \times 10^{-3})$	US no.	Tyler no.
1.	22.6		7/8 in.	0.883 in.
2.	16.0	16	5/8 in.	0.624 in.
3.	11.2	11.2	7/16 in.	0.441 in.
4.	8.0	8.00	5/16 in.	2 1/2 mesh
5.	5.66	5.66	No. 3 1/2	3 1/2 mesh
6.	4.00	4.00	5	5 mesh
7.	2.83	2.80	7	7 mesh
8.	2.00	2.00	10	9 mesh
9.	1.41	1.41	14	12 mesh
10.	1.00	1.00	18	16 mesh
11.	0.71	0.710	25	24 mesh
12.	0.500	0.500	35	32 mesh
13.	0.354	0.355	45	42 mesh
14.	0.250	0.250	60	60 mesh
15.	0.177	0.180	80	80 mesh
16.	0.125	0.125	120	115 mesh
17.	0.088	0.090	170	170 mesh
18.	0.063	0.063	230	250 mesh
19.	0.044	0.045	325	325 mesh

*Note: 0.50 m $\times 10^{-3}$ aperture = 35 US No. = 32 mesh

Index